全国高等教育药学类规划教材

# 药物化学实验

## 双语教程

## Experiments of Medicinal Chemistry

李　雯　刘宏民　主编

尤启冬　主审

U0196426

化学工业出版社

·北京·

《药物化学实验双语教程（Experiments of Medicinal Chemistry）》按照从基础操作到综合实验的顺序安排了 10 个经典化学药物合成实验，强调了药物化学理论教学与实验的关联，关注学生实验能力和科研素质的培养。附录包含实验报告模板、常规仪器和思考题参考答案三部分内容。

《药物化学实验双语教程（Experiments of Medicinal Chemistry）》可作为高等医药院校药学类专业学生（包括留学生）的实验教材，也可供其他药学相关专业从业人员参考使用。

**图书在版编目（CIP）数据**

药物化学实验双语教程＝Experiments of Medicinal Chemistry：汉英对照/李雯，刘宏民主编.—北京：化学工业出版社，2019.9

全国高等教育药学类规划教材
ISBN 978-7-122-34698-8

Ⅰ.①药⋯　Ⅱ.①李⋯ ②刘⋯　Ⅲ.①药物化学-化学实验-高等学校-教材-汉、英　Ⅳ.①R914-33

中国版本图书馆 CIP 数据核字（2019）第 120286 号

责任编辑：褚红喜　　　　　　　　　　　　　装帧设计：关　飞
责任校对：杜杏然

出版发行：化学工业出版社（北京市东城区青年湖南街 13 号　邮政编码 100011）
印　　装：三河市双峰印刷装订有限公司
787mm×1092mm　1/16　印张 9½　彩插 3　字数 227 千字　　2019 年 9 月北京第 1 版第 1 次印刷

购书咨询：010-64518888　　售后服务：010-64518899
网　　址：http://www.cip.com.cn
凡购买本书，如有缺损质量问题，本社销售中心负责调换。

定　　价：29.80 元　　　　　　　　　　　　　　　　　版权所有　违者必究

# Experiments of Medicinal Chemistry

### Editor in chief

**Wen Li** (School of pharmaceutical sciences, Zhengzhou University)

**Hongmin Liu** (School of pharmaceutical sciences, Zhengzhou University)

### Reviewer in chief

**Qidong You** (School of pharmacy, China Pharmaceutical University)

### Editors

**Lina Ding** (School of pharmaceutical sciences, Zhengzhou University)

**En Zhang** (School of pharmaceutical sciences, Zhengzhou University)

**Yajing Chen** (School of pharmaceutical sciences, Zhengzhou University)

**Yichao Zheng** (School of pharmaceutical sciences, Zhengzhou University)

**Qiurong Zhang** (School of pharmaceutical sciences, Zhengzhou University)

# 《药物化学实验双语教程》 编写组

## 主 编

李 雯 （郑州大学药学院）

刘宏民 （郑州大学药学院）

## 主 审

尤启冬 （中国药科大学药学院）

## 编 者

丁丽娜 （郑州大学药学院）

张 恩 （郑州大学药学院）

陈亚静 （郑州大学药学院）

郑一超 （郑州大学药学院）

张秋荣 （郑州大学药学院）

# 序

随着我国教育国际化进程的发展，高等教育的国际化已由原有的单纯"走出去"，逐渐转变为"走出去"和"招进来"相结合的模式。越来越多的外国留学生，特别是"一带一路"沿线国家和亚非等国的外国留学生到中国来学习。但我国双语教材的建设速度与日益增多的留学生发展趋势不能同步，因此，进行双语教材的编写和推广使用工作有着非常重要的价值和意义。

郑州大学药学院根据药学专业中国学生双语教学的需求和留学生教学的需求，开展实验教学研究，编写和出版了《药物化学实验双语教程（Experiments of Medicinal Chemistry）》。

该教材重视加强学生科研能力的培养，是作者针对国内学生和留学生的实际情况，分析现行各版本教材的内容和特点，博采众家所长而编写的教材，具有以下特色：

（1）在实验原理部分，增加主要原料和产物的物性常数，包括分子量、熔点、沸点和溶解度等参数，以培养学生通过思考和实验操作，触类旁通，提高解决问题的能力，且配以图表便于理解。

（2）增加安全提醒内容，以预防部分学生对危险化学品的错误使用而造成严重后果。

（3）在实验操作方面，增加实验装置图示，以方便学生以直观的方式尽快理解实验操作过程。

（4）增加药物受体和配体相互作用的计算机模拟图示，体现了实验课程对理论课程知识的综合应用和拓展。

（5）为培养学生对实验现象规范记录和结果分析能力，本教材提供了实例并提出了具体的要求，使学生进一步联系理论，做出分析比较。

（6）增加思考题的参考答案，给学生一些提示，方便更好地理解实验相关问题，有助于培养学生的学习兴趣。

相信本教材的出版能够促进我国药物化学实验双语教学的发展。

尤启冬

（国家实验教学示范中心联席会药学学科组组长、国家教学名师）

2019 年 3 月

# 前　言

为适应我国本科教学国际化的发展趋势，根据药物化学实验课程的基本要求，结合我们多年的教学经验和科研工作，编写了这本《药物化学实验双语教程（Experiments of Medicinal Chemistry)》。

本书包括 10 个化学药物合成实验，实验一至实验八为我们多年药物化学实验教学实践的总结，实验九和实验十为编者科研工作的结果。在化学药物合成实验的安排上，本书按照从基础操作到综合实验的顺序进行编写；在内容上，本书不仅给出了实验原理、操作过程、注意事项和思考题，而且给出了药物分子和靶标的作用机制图示、主要原料和中间体的物理常数、实验装置、安全提示和思考题参考答案。旨在强调药物化学理论教学与实验的关联，关注学生实验能力和科研素质培养。10 个化学药物合成实验的难易程度和实验学时有明显的区分度，可满足不同专业和不同层次学生的教学需求。

本教材的实验一、实验二、实验七、实验九由李雯、刘宏民编写，实验三、实验四由陈亚静编写，实验五由丁丽娜编写，实验六由张恩编写，实验八由郑一超编写，实验十由张秋荣编写，全书由尤启冬教授审订。书中药物分子和靶标的作用机制部分由丁丽娜及其研究生阎影、马超亚、王志正、高琦冰、孙旭东和杨晶等借助 MOE 软件进行模拟研究编写而成。留学中国的博士研究生 Moges Dessale Asmamaw、研究生常英杰、李瑞鹏及本科生朱林元参与了本书的语言润色工作。药物化学实验双语教材的建设，任重而道远。

《药物化学实验双语教程（Experiments of Medicinal Chemistry)》采用中英双语体系编写，可作为普通高等医药院校药学类各专业学生（包括留学生）的实验教材，也可供其他药学相关专业师生参考使用。

编者
2019 年 3 月

# Preface

In order to adapt to the development trend of internationalization of undergraduate teaching in our country, according to the basic requirements of pharmaceutical chemistry experiment course combined with our years of teaching experience and scientific research work, this "bilingual course of pharmaceutical chemistry experiment" has been compiled.

In this textbook, 10 synthetic experiments of chemical drugs are included. Experiments 1 through 8 are the summaries of many years teaching practices, Experiments 9 and 10 are the results of the editors' scientific research work. They are arranged by the order from basic to comprehensive gradually. In each experiment, more than the experiment principle, operation process, notes and discussion questions are given, the action mechanism diagrams of drug molecule and target, physical constants of key raw materials and intermediates, experimental equipments, safety tips and reference answers of discussion questions are described. This textbook emphasizes the relationship between theoretical teaching and experiment of pharmaceutical chemistry, and pays attention to the cultivation of students' experimental ability and scientific research quality. There is a clear distinction between the difficulty and time of 10 experiments to meet the teaching needs of students from different majors and levels.

Experiments 1, 2, 7 and 9 of this textbook were written by Wen Li and Hongmin Liu, Experiments 3 and 4 by Yajing Chen, Experiment 5 by Lina Ding, Experiment 6 by En Zhang, Experiment 8 by Yichao Zheng and Experiment 10 by Qiurong Zhang. This textbook was revised by Professor Qidong You. The mechanistic studies between the drug molecule and the corresponding target were investigated and written by Lina Ding and her graduate students Ying Yan, Chaoya Ma, Zhizheng Wang, Qibing Gao, Xudong Sun and Jing Yang with the help of MOE software. We appreciate the foreign PhD student Moges Dessale Asmamaw, graduate students Yingjie Chang, Ruipeng Li and undergraduate student Linyuan Zhu who involved in the language correction of this textbook. The construction of bilingual textbooks is on the developing way.

This textbook is compiled in a Chinese-English bilingual system and can be used in the experimental teaching of pharmaceutical students (including foreign students) in medical colleges and universities.

**Editors**
**March 2019**

# Contents
# 目 录

# Experiment 1

# Recrystallization of Acetanilide

## Background

Acetanilide (Fig. 1-1) has an odourless solid chemical of leaf or flake-like appearance. It is also known as $N$-phenylacetamide, acetanil, or acetanilid, and was formerly known as the trade name Antifebrin.

Acetanilide was the first aniline derivative which was found to possess analgesic and antipyretic properties, and was quickly introduced into the medical practice by A. Cahn and P. Hepp in 1886. But due to the unacceptable toxic effects, it has been replaced by a new generation of acetyl drugs such as Phenacetin and Paracetamol (Fig. 1-1).

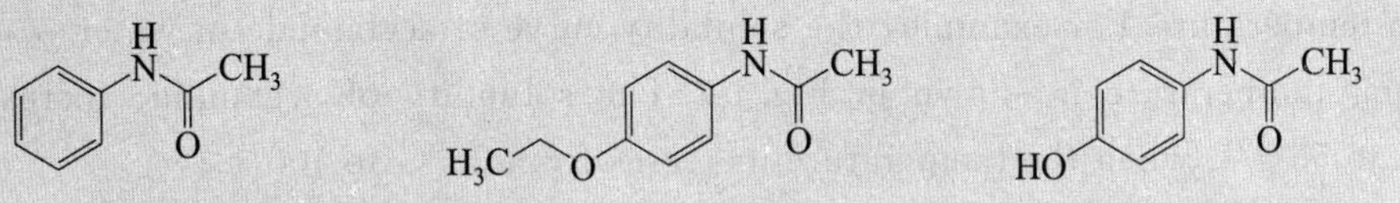

Fig. 1-1 Chemical structures of Acetanilide, Phenacetin and Paracetamol

Now, Acetanilide is mainly used as industrial rubber vulcanization promoters, stabilizers of fiber fat coatings, stabilizers of hydrogen peroxide and for the synthesis of camphor.

Acetanilide belongs to non-steroidal anti-inflammatory drug (NSAIDs) which general target the cyclooxygenase and lipoxygenase enzymes. The possible binding mode of acetanilide with cyclooxygenase 2 (COX-2) (PDB: 5F1A) is illustrated by **Color Diagram 1.** The acetyl group in the acetanilide forms a hydrogen bond with the oxygen of the hydroxy in the Ser 530 side chain and the benzene ring forms hydrophobic interactions with the surrounding hydrophobic residues.

## Ⅰ Purposes and Requirements

1. To master the recrystallization principle.
2. To master the operation of recrystallization.
3. To understand the interaction between acetanilide and target.

## Ⅱ Experimental Principle

### 1. Physical data of the main reactants and product

| Name | Structure /CAS No. | Formula /M. Wt | b. p. or m. p. /℃ | Solubility/(g/L) |
|------|------|------|------|------|
| Acetanilide | (structure) 103-84-4 | $C_8H_9NO$ 135. 16 | m. p. 113~115 | In water: 5. 5 (at 100 ℃) and 0. 46 (at 20 ℃) In ethanol: 36. 9 (at 20 ℃) In methanol: 69. 5 (at 20 ℃) In chloroform: 3. 6 (at 20 ℃) |

### 2. Recrystallization principle

Compounds obtained from reaction mixtures always contain some impurities. The impurities may include some residues of soluble, insoluble and colored compounds. To obtain a pure product, these impurities must be completely removed.

Recrystallization is the primary method for purifying solid organic compounds. The principle of recrystallization is that the amount of solute that can be dissolved in a solvent increases with temperature. For example, the solubility curve of acetanilide in water with respect to varying temperature is shown in Fig. 1-2. The solubility of acetanilide increases from 4. 6 g/L to 55 g/L when the temperature increases from 20 ℃ to 100 ℃.

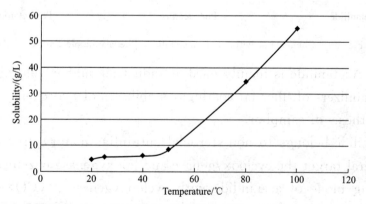

Fig. 1-2   Solubility curve of acetanilide in water

In a recrystallization procedure (Fig. 1-3), selection of an appropriate solvent is the most important factor. When an appropriate solvent is selected, solid compounds which contain some impurities can dissolve in the solvent at or near their boiling points. The insoluble impurities can be removed by hot filtration. This step of recrystallization should be conducted

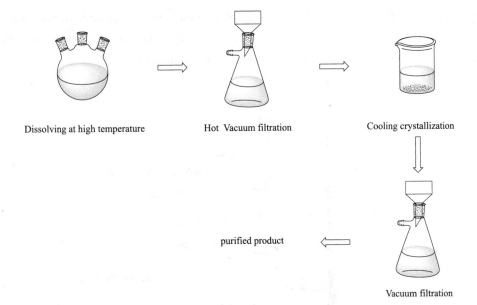

Dissolving at high temperature        Hot  Vacuum filtration        Cooling crystallization

purified product        Vacuum filtration

Fig. 1-3　Procedure of recrystallization

while keeping the filtration set-up hot so as to prevent premature crystal formation. Next, allow the hot solution to cool down to the room temperature before collecting the purified crystals by filtration. Note that the soluble impurities will remain in the filtrate.

The boiling points and dielectric constants of the commonly used solvents are summarized in Table 1-1 below.

Table 1-1　The boiling point and dielectric constant of the commonly used solvents

| Solvent | b. p. /℃ | Dielectric Constant* | Solvent | b. p. /℃ | Dielectric Constant* |
|---|---|---|---|---|---|
| N-Methylformamide | 183 | 182. 4 | Tetrahydrofuran | 66 | 7. 6 |
| Water | 100 | 78. 4 | Ethyl acetate | 78 | 6. 0 |
| Dimethylsulfoxide | 189 | 46. 5 | Chloroform | 61. 2 | 4. 8 |
| N,N-Dimethyl-formamide | 153 | 36. 7 | Diethylether | 34. 4 | 4. 2 |
| Methanol | 64. 5 | 32. 7 | Toluene | 110. 6 | 2. 4 |
| Ethanol | 78 | 24. 5 | Cyclohexane | 81 | 1. 9 |
| Acetone | 56 | 20. 6 | n-Heptane | 98. 4 | 1. 9 |
| 2-Methyl-2-propanol, t-Butanol | 82. 3 | 12. 5 | n-Hexane | 68. 7 | 1. 9 |
| 1,2-Dichloroethane | 83. 5 | 10. 4 | n-Pentane | 36. 1 | 1. 8 |
| Dichloromethane | 39. 6 | 8. 9 | | | |

* The dielectric constant is a measure of the solvent's ability to separate ions. In general, ionic compounds are more soluble in solvents with high dielectric constants.

## Ⅲ  Experimental Equipments and Raw Materials

### 1. Experimental equipments

Dissolving set-up is shown in Fig. 1-4. This experimental set-up is composed from three-neck round-bottom flask, spherical condenser tube, magnetic stirrer and thermometer.

Vacuum filtration set-up is shown in Fig. 1-5. This experimental set-up is composed from filter flask, Buchner funnel, filter paper and vacuum pump.

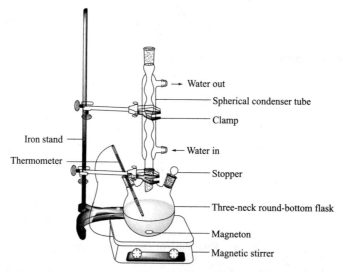

Fig. 1-4　Dissolving set-up

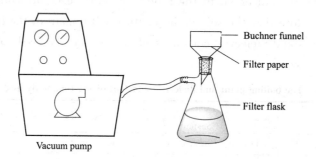

Fig. 1-5　Vacuum filtration set-up

## 2. Raw materials

| Name | Quantity | Quality | Use |
| --- | --- | --- | --- |
| Acetanilide | 2 g (0. 015 mol) | Industrial grade | Raw material |
| Activated carbon (Charcoal) | 0. 5 g | — | Decolorizing substance |
| Distilled water | 40 mL | — | Recrystallization solvent |

## Ⅳ　Operations

（1）Equip the dissolving set-up as shown in Fig. 1-4. Add 2 g of the impure acetanilide and 40 mL of distilled water into the 100 mL three-neck round-bottom flask. Dissolve the solute completely by stirring （magnetic stirrer） and heating up the mixture to 100 ℃.

（2）Once acetanilide is dissolved completely, slightly cool down the solution to about 95 ℃ followed by the addition of 0. 5 g of activated carbon. Decolorization is achieved by heating the mixture for about 10 minutes for gentle refluxing.

(3) Equip the vacuum filtration set-up as shown in Fig. 1-5. Filter the hot solution by vacuum filtration. Allow the filtrate to cool down to room temperature in an ice-water bath for about 10 minutes. Caution should be taken not shaking or stirring the filtrate.

(4) The pure product is collected by filtrating again. Attention should be paid to drain the solvent as far as possible.

(5) The product is dried under infrared lamp. Weigh the pure product, calculate the yield and measure the melting point.

(6) Send the final product to the place where the guide teachers designated.

## V Experimental Results

### 1. Yield
Calculate the percent yield of acetanilide.

$$\text{Yield} = \frac{\text{Practical production}}{\text{Theoretical production}} \times 100\% = \frac{(\quad)}{2 \text{ g}} \times 100\% = (\quad)\%$$

### 2. Appearance and melting point of the pure product
A. Appearance: _____ ;

B. m. p. :

  Theoretical value: 113~115 ℃;

  Practical value: _____ .

### 3. Analysis of experimental results

_____
_____
_____
_____
_____
_____
_____
_____ .

## VI Notes

1. In general, the amount of activated carbon is $1\% \sim 5\%$ (by weight) of the crude product according to the color depth.

2. Adding activated carbon while the solution is boiling can easily cause serious bumping. Therefore, when the activated carbon is added, the temperature of the solution must be slightly lower.

3. The filtrate of the hot solution should be allowed to cool slowly to room temperature. Gradual cooling is conducive to the formation of large well-defined crystals.

4. When the crystals are collected and washed, allow the water pump to run for several

minutes so that the crystals have an opportunity to dry.

# VII Discussion Questions

1. Why the activated carbon can not be added to the boiling solution when it used as a decolorizing agent?

2. What are the commonly used recrystallization solvents?

(By Wen Li，Hongmin Liu)

# 乙酰苯胺重结晶

## 背景知识

乙酰苯胺（Acetanilide）为无味，白色叶状或片状结晶（图 1-1）。也称作 *N*-苯基乙酰胺，曾以商品名退热冰应用于临床。

乙酰苯胺是第一个被发现的具有镇痛和解热作用的苯胺类衍生物，1886 年，A. Cahn 和 P. Hepp 将其应用于临床。但是，乙酰苯胺具有严重的副作用从而被新一代的乙酰苯胺类药物取代，比如非那西汀和对乙酰氨基酚。

乙酰苯胺　　　　　　　　非那西汀　　　　　　　对乙酰氨基酚

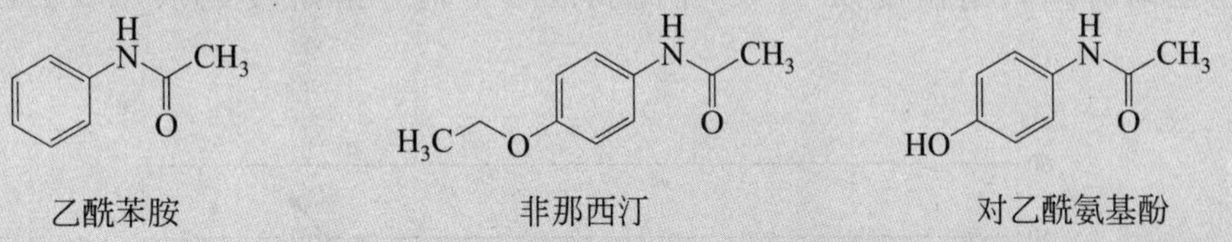

图 1-1　乙酰苯胺、非那西汀和对乙酰氨基酚的化学结构式

目前，乙酰苯胺主要用作工业橡胶硫化促进剂、纤维脂肪涂层稳定剂、双氧水稳定剂和合成樟脑。

乙酰苯胺属于非甾体抗炎药，通常这类药物的作用靶点为环氧合酶和脂氧合酶。**彩插 1** 给出了乙酰苯胺和环氧合酶-2（COX-2）可能的结合方式模型，蛋白晶体结构为 PDB：5F1A，分子模拟结果显示乙酰苯胺可以与水杨酸结合位点形成良好的相互作用。乙酰苯胺在此位点的作用模式以及结合口袋的表面图分别如**彩插 1**（A）、（B）所示。（乙酰苯胺中乙酰基部分的羰基氧与 Ser 530 侧链的羟基形成氢键，苯环与周围的氨基酸形成疏水作用）

## Ⅰ　目的与要求

1. 掌握重结晶原理。
2. 掌握重结晶操作。
3. 了解乙酰苯胺与靶标的作用方式。

## Ⅱ 实验原理

### 1. 主要反应物和产物的物理常数

| 名称 | 结构式<br>/CAS 号 | 分子式<br>/分子量 | 沸点或熔点<br>/℃ | 溶解度/(g/L) |
|------|------|------|------|------|
| 乙酰苯胺 | （结构式）<br>103-84-4 | $C_8H_9NO$<br>135.16 | m. p.<br>113～115 | 水：55（100 ℃），4.6（20 ℃）；<br>乙醇：36.9（20 ℃）；<br>甲醇：69.5（20 ℃）；<br>氯仿：3.6（20 ℃） |

### 2. 重结晶原理

反应获得的化合物往往含有一些杂质，这些杂质可以是可溶的，不易溶解的和有色的化合物。若要获得纯净的化合物，必须除去以上所述及的杂质。重结晶是除去固体化合物杂质的常用方法之一。

重结晶的原理是：一般情况下，溶质在溶液中的溶解度随着温度的升高而增大。例如，图 1-2 给出了乙酰苯胺在水中的溶解度曲线，在水中，乙酰苯胺随着温度的升高其溶解度也逐渐升高，当温度从 20 ℃ 升高到 100 ℃ 时，溶解度则从 4.6 g/L 增大至 55 g/L。

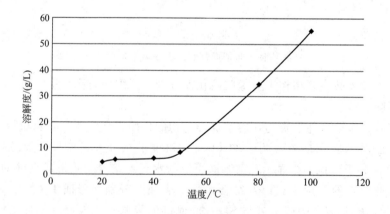

图 1-2　乙酰苯胺在水中的溶解度曲线

图 1-3 为重结晶操作的一般过程。首先，选择适宜的重结晶溶剂，使含有杂质的固体化合物溶于溶剂或者在接近沸点时溶于溶剂，然后，通过热过滤除去不溶性杂质。热过滤过程中要先将过滤装置预热以防止过早析出晶体而无法过滤。随后，在热的滤液逐渐冷却的过程中，重结晶后析出纯的晶体，过滤收集纯化后的产物，而可溶性杂质留在滤液中。

重结晶溶剂的选取是非常重要的因素。常用的重结晶溶剂的沸点和介电常数汇总于表 1-1。

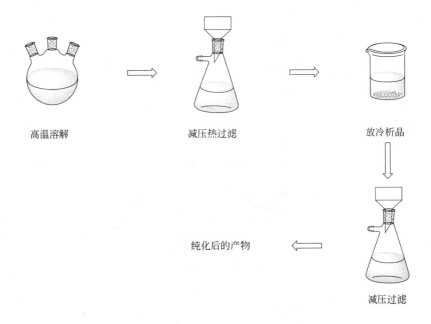

图 1-3  重结晶操作的一般过程

表 1-1  常用重结晶溶剂沸点和介电常数汇总

| 溶剂 | 沸点/℃ | 介电常数* | 溶剂 | 沸点/℃ | 介电常数* |
|---|---|---|---|---|---|
| N-甲基甲酰胺 | 183 | 182.4 | 四氢呋喃 | 66 | 7.6 |
| 水 | 100 | 78.4 | 乙酸乙酯 | 78 | 6.0 |
| 二甲基亚砜 | 189 | 46.5 | 氯仿 | 61.2 | 4.8 |
| N,N-二甲基甲酰胺 | 153 | 36.7 | 乙醚 | 34.4 | 4.2 |
| 甲醇 | 64.5 | 32.7 | 甲苯 | 110.6 | 2.4 |
| 乙醇 | 78 | 24.5 | 环己烷 | 81 | 1.9 |
| 丙酮 | 56 | 20.6 | n-庚烷 | 98.4 | 1.9 |
| 2-甲基-2-丙醇,叔丁醇 | 82.3 | 12.5 | n-己烷 | 68.7 | 1.9 |
| 1,2-二氯乙烷 | 83.5 | 10.4 | n-戊烷 | 36.1 | 1.8 |
| 二氯甲烷 | 39.6 | 8.9 | | | |

* 介电常数是衡量溶剂的解离离子能力的量度。一般情况下，离子化合物更容易溶于高介电常数的溶剂中。

## Ⅲ  实验装置和原料

### 1. 实验装置

溶解装置见图 1-4，该实验装置由三颈烧瓶、球形冷凝管、磁力搅拌器、温度计等组成。

抽滤装置见图 1-5，该装置由抽滤瓶、布氏漏斗、滤纸和真空泵组成。

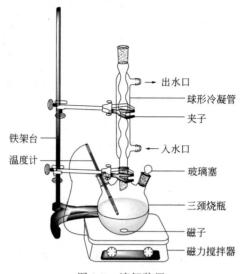

出水口
球形冷凝管
夹子
铁架台
温度计
入水口
玻璃塞
三颈烧瓶
磁子
磁力搅拌器

图 1-4　溶解装置

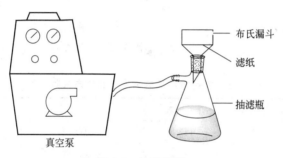

布氏漏斗
滤纸
抽滤瓶
真空泵

图 1-5　抽滤装置

**2. 原料**

| 名称 | 用量 | 试剂级别 | 用途 |
|---|---|---|---|
| 乙酰苯胺 | 2 g（0.015 mol） | 工业级 | 原料 |
| 活性炭 | 0.5 g | — | 脱色剂 |
| 蒸馏水 | 40 mL | — | 重结晶溶剂 |

## Ⅳ 实验操作

（1）在 100 mL 三颈烧瓶中，加入 2 g 乙酰苯胺粗品、40 mL 蒸馏水，按照图 1-4 搭建溶解装置。边搅拌边升高温度至 100 ℃。

（2）溶解完全后，降温至 95 ℃，加入 0.5 g 活性炭。然后，加热至沸腾，并保持 10 min，脱色。

（3）采用图 1-5 的真空抽滤装置进行热过滤，滤液静置放冷至室温，然后冰水浴 10 min，析出晶体。注意不要振摇或搅拌滤液。

（4）过滤沉淀，尽量抽干。

（5）产品置于红外灯下干燥，称重，计算收率，测熔点。

（6）将产物送到指导教师指定的产品回收处。

## V 实验结果

### 1. 收率
按下式计算乙酰苯胺的收率。

$$收率 = \frac{产品实际产量}{产品理论产量} \times 100\% = \frac{(\quad)}{2\,g} \times 100\% = (\quad)\%$$

### 2. 产品外观与熔点
A. 外观：_____；

B. 熔点：

理论值：113～115 ℃；

实测值：_____。

### 3. 实验结果分析
_____
_____
_____
_____
_____
_____
_____
_____。

## VI 注意事项

1. 一般情况下，根据粗品颜色的深浅程度，活性炭的用量为粗品质量的 1%～5%。

2. 当溶液沸腾时，加入活性炭易引起暴沸，因此，加入活性炭时，需要将溶液稍微降温。

3. 经热过滤所获得的滤液，在降温至室温的过程中，需要缓慢降温。缓慢降温是获得较大粒度、完好晶体的关键因素。

4. 当晶体过滤和洗涤后，应让真空泵继续抽气几分钟，以使得获得的晶体尽可能干燥。

## VII 思考题

1. 作为脱色剂，活性炭为什么不能在沸腾时加入溶液中？

2. 常用的重结晶溶剂有哪些？

（李雯　刘宏民）

# Experiment 2
# Synthesis of Aspirin

## Background

Salicylic acid was isolated from the willow bark tree in 1823 and its chemical structure is defined by the medicinal chemists (Fig. 2-1). Since then, salicylic acid is widely used in the clinical practice as anti-rheumatic and antipyretic analgesic drug. But, it has an apparent stomach stimulating effects which can induce gastrointestinal discomfort and peptic ulcer disease among others.

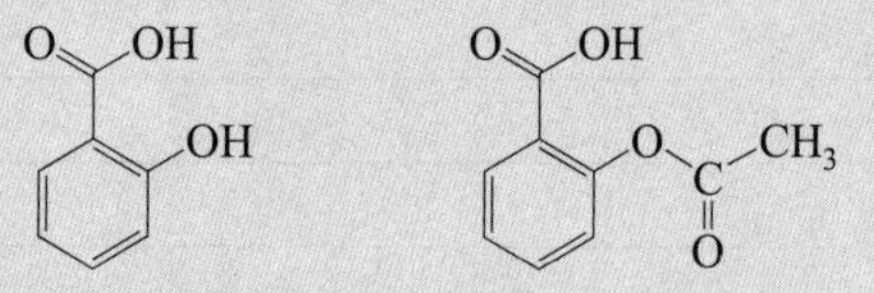

Salicylic acid            Aspirin
                    (2- acetyloxy benzoic acid)

Fig. 2-1   Chemical structure of
Salicylic acid and Aspirin

Aspirin is derived from salicylic acid by substituting the phenolic hydroxy group on benzene cycle with acetoxyl group (Fig. 2-1). Aspirin has a much lower side effect than salicylic acid. In addition, the structural modification also extends the clinical use of aspirin to anti-thrombosis which exhibits beneficial effects in the prevention and treatment of cardiovascular diseases, such as coronary heart disease and atherosclerosis.

Aspirin belongs to non-steroidal anti-inflammatory drug (NSAIDs). Aspirin for anti-inflammatory treatment principle is via the loops of aspirin and cyclooxygenase 2 (COX-2) (**Color Diagram 2**). The composite crystal structure of the cyclooxygenase COX-2 and salicylic acid (PDB: 5F1A) can be used to determine the binding mode of aspirin. The binding mode aspirin with COX-2 and the surface of the pocket are shown in **Color Diagram 2**. There is a hydrogen bond formed between the carbonyl oxygen in the acetyl group in aspirin and the phenol oxygen in Tyr 385, as well as the carboxyl group of the carboxyl group forms the hydrogen bond with the hydroxy oxygen of the Ser 530. The benzene ring is surrounded by the hydrophobic side chains.

# I Purposes and Requirements

1. To master the acetylation reaction and its use on structural modification of drug substances.

2. To master the anhydrous operation method, and the use of coloration reaction on the end-poinl determination of organic synthesis.

3. To understand the interaction between aspirin and target.

# II Principle of the Reaction

## 1. Physical data of the main reactants and product

| Name | Structure /CAS No. | Formula /M. Wt | b. p. or m. p. /°C | Solubility |
|------|-----|-----|-----|-----|
| Salicylic acid | 69-72-7 | $C_7H_6O_3$ 138. 12 | m. p. 158~161 | In water: 1. 8 g/L (at 20 °C) In ethanol: 1 mol/L (at 20 °C) |
| Acetic anhydride | 108-24-7 | $C_4H_6O_3$ 102. 09 | b. p. 138~139 | Reaction with water to form acetic acid; and miscible with ether, chloroform and benzene |
| Aspirin | 50-78-2 | $C_9H_8O_4$ 180. 16 | m. p. 135~138 | In water: 3. 3 g/L (at 20 °C) In DMSO: 100 mmol/L (at 20 °C) |

## 2. Synthetic Route

Salicylic acid     Acetic anhydride     Aspirin     Acetic acid

Aspirin is synthesized by an acylation reaction using salicylic acid and acetic anhydride as starting materials. The reaction is catalyzied by concentrated sulfuric acid and should take place in an anhydrous environment.

**Safety Tips:** The acetical anhydride and sulfuric acid can cause bad burns and thus will be used in the hood. If they come in contact with your skin, wash the area immediately with copious amounts of water.

# Ⅲ Experimental Equipments and Raw Materials

## 1. Experimental equipments

Reaction experimental set-up is shown in Fig. 2-2. This experimental set-up is composed from three-neck round-bottom flask，spherical condenser tube，magnetic stirrer and thermometer.

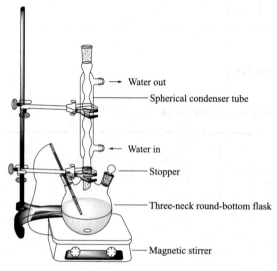

Fig. 2-2　Reaction experimental set-up

Vacuum filtration experimental set-up，Fig. 2-3，is composed from filter flask，Buchner funnel，filter paper and vacuum pump.

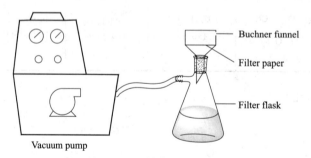

Fig. 2-3　Vacuum filtration experimental set-up

## 2. Raw materials

| Name | Quantity | Quality | Use |
| --- | --- | --- | --- |
| Salicyclic acid | 8. 3 g (0. 06 mol) | C. P. | Reactant |
| Acetic anhydride | 15 mL (0. 159 mol) | C. P. | Acetylating agent |
| Sulfuric acid | 0. 4 mL (5 drops) | C. P. | Catalyst |
| $FeCl_3$ reagent | 1 drop | — | End point indicator |
| Ethanol | 12 mL | 95% | Solvent for recryst |
| $H_2O$ | Proper amount | — | Solvent |
| Active carbon (Charcoal) | 0. 5 g | — | Decolorizing substance |

# Ⅳ Operations

## 1. Synthesis of aspirin crude product

（1）Equip the reaction experimental set-up as shown in Fig. 2-2. Add 15 mL of acetic anhydride and 5 drops of concentrated sulfuric acid into the 100 mL three-neck round-bottom flask. Heat the solution to 55~60 ℃ while stirring with a magnetic stirrer.

（2）Keeping the solution at 55~60 ℃ and add 8.3 g of salicylic acid to the reaction flask. The white crystals can be observed to dissolve gradually with stirring.

（3）Endpoint detection. One drop of reaction solution is taken out and put into the reaction board. The reaction solution should be changed to yellow upon addition of one drop of $FeCl_3$ reagent. The reaction solution should not show violet. If the solution shows light violet, then the reaction needs to be continued.

（4）If the reaction reachs the endpoint, cool the flask to room temperature and then put into a cold water-bath. Add 75 mL of water to the flask and collect the product by vacuum filtration. （Vacuum filtration experimental set-up is shown in Fig. 2-3）.

（5）Wash the product in 2~3 times with ice water. Attention should be paid to drain the solvent as far as possible.

（6）Dry the product under infrared lamp and measure the weight.

## 2. Recrystallization of aspirin

（1）Equip the experimental set-up as shown in Fig. 2-2. Add the crude product （aspirin） and 12 mL ethanol into the 100 mL three-neck round-bottom flask. Dissolve the solute completely by stirring （magnetic stirrer） and heat the mixture up to 50 ℃.

（2）Once the crude product （aspirin） is dissolved completely, 0.5 g of activated carbon （decolorizing substance） is added to the reaction mixture at 50 ℃. Then, the mixture is kept at 50 ℃ for 5 minutes to decolorize the product.

（3）Equip the vacuum filtration experimental set-up as shown in Fig. 2-3. Filter the hot solution by vacuum filtration. Allow the filtrate to cool down to room temperature （just put the filtrate on the experiment table）. Add 12 mL of cold distilled water to the filtrate and collect the pure product by filtering again.

（4）Wash the pure product 2~3 times with 30% ethanol. Attention should be paid to drain the solvent as far as possible.

（5）The product is dried under infrared lamp. Weigh the pure product, calculate the yield and measure the melting point.

（6）Send the final product to the place where the guide teachers designated.

# Ⅴ Experimental Results

## 1. Yield

（1）Calculate the theoretical production of aspirin

Salicyclic acid —————— Aspirin

$$M_w = 138.12 \text{ g/mol} \text{———}M_w = 180.16 \text{ g/mol}$$

$$0.06 \text{ mol} \text{———} 0.06 \text{ mol}$$

Theoretical production $= 0.6 \text{ mol} \times 180.16 \text{ g/mol} = 10.81 \text{ g}$

（2）Calculate the percent yield of aspirin

$$\text{Yield} = \frac{\text{Practical production}}{\text{Theoretical production}} \times 100\% = \frac{(\quad)}{10.81 \text{ g}} \times 100\% = (\quad)\%$$

## 2. Appearance and melting point of product

A. Appearance: _____ ;

B. m. p. :

　　Theoretical value: 135～138 ℃ ;

　　Practical value: _____ .

## 3. Analysis of experimental results

_____
_____
_____
_____
_____
_____
_____ .

# Ⅵ Notes

1. During the synthesis of the crude product, the anhydrous condition is the first decisive factor. The reason is that acetic anhydride can be decomposed by moist air or water. So, all apparatus and raw materials should be absolutely dried.

2. Controlling the reaction temperature is the second decisive factor. This is due to the fact that when the reaction temperature is above 60 ℃, salicylic acid will be oxidized by $H_2SO_4$ (a strong oxidizing agent) and it will change into yellow or dark oxidized product. So, the reaction and the recrystallization temperature must be controlled below 60 ℃.

# Ⅶ Discussion Questions

1. Structurally, why dose/might our room smell like vinegar during this experiment?

2. Structurally, why salicylic and acetylsalicylic acid are considered as acids?

（By Wen Li, Hongmin Liu）

# 实验二

# 阿司匹林的合成

## 背景知识

1823 年，药物化学家从柳树皮中分离获得了水杨酸，并确证其化学结构（图 2-1）。此后，水杨酸作为抗风湿和解热镇痛药物被广泛应用。然而，水杨酸具有明显的胃刺激作用，可引起胃不适症状和消化性溃疡等副作用。

当把水杨酸的酚羟基酰化为乙酰氧基，便得到了阿司匹林（图 2-1）。阿司匹林的副作用比水杨酸降低很多。而且，阿司匹林的临床应用还扩展到了抗血栓形成，对冠心病、动脉粥样硬化等心血管疾病的防治也有积极作用（图 2-1）。

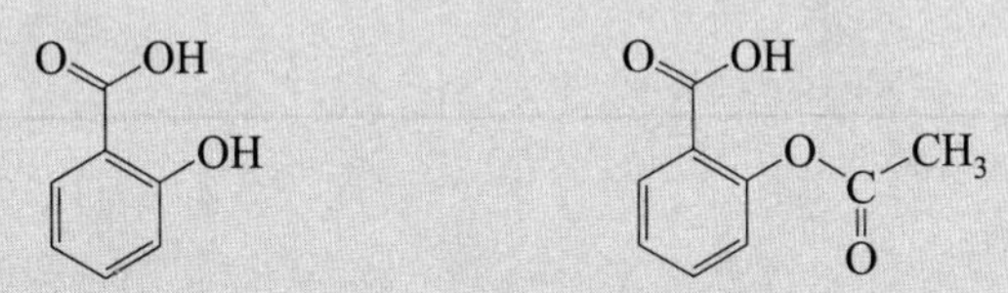

水杨酸

阿司匹林
(2-乙酰氧基水杨酸)

图 2-1　水杨酸和阿司匹林化学结构式

阿司匹林属于非甾体抗炎药，**彩插 2** 模拟了阿司匹林与环氧合酶-2（COX-2）的结合模式图，其中蛋白晶体结构为 PDB：5F1A。阿司匹林与水杨酸在和 COX-2 作用时，作用位点相似，阿司匹林在此位点的作用模式以及结合口袋的表面图如**彩插 2** 所示。（阿司匹林中乙酰基部分的羰基氧与 Tyr 385 的酚氧形成氢键，苯环与周围的侧链形成疏水作用，羧基部分的羰基氧与 Ser 530 的羟基氧形成氢键。）

## I　目的与要求

1. 掌握酯化反应原理和其在药物结构修饰中的应用。
2. 掌握无水反应操作，掌握颜色反应在反应终点判断方面的应用。
3. 了解阿司匹林与靶标的作用方式。

## Ⅱ 实验原理

### 1. 主要反应物和产物的物理常数

| 名称 | 结构式 /CAS 号 | 分子式 /分子量 | 沸点或熔点/℃ | 溶解度 |
|---|---|---|---|---|
| 水杨酸 | 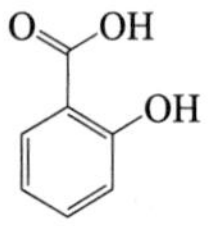 69-72-7 | $C_7H_6O_3$ 138.12 | m. p. 158~161 | 水：1.8 g/L（20 ℃）；乙醇：1 mol/L（20 ℃） |
| 乙酸酐 | 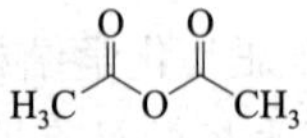 108-24-7 | $C_4H_6O_3$ 102.09 | b. p. 138~139 | 遇水反应，生成醋酸；易溶于乙醚、氯仿和苯 |
| 阿司匹林 | 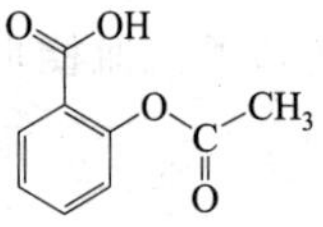 50-78-2 | $C_9H_8O_4$ 180.16 | m. p. 135~138 | 水：3.3 g/L（20 ℃）；DMSO：100 mmol/L（20 ℃） |

### 2. 合成路线

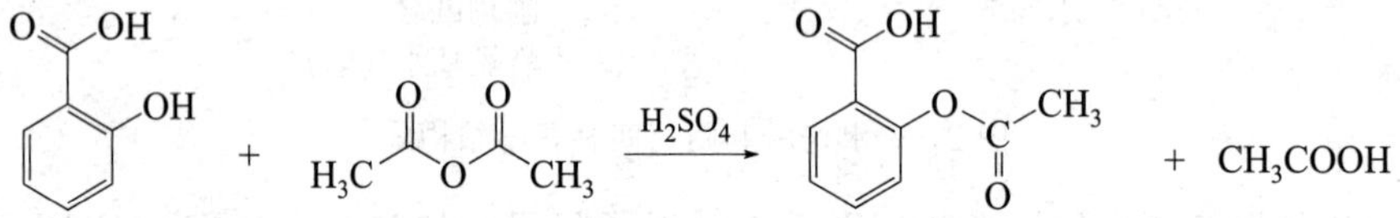

水杨酸　　　　　　　醋酸酐　　　　　　　阿司匹林　　　　醋酸

水杨酸与醋酸酐在浓硫酸催化下，发生酰化反应生成阿司匹林和醋酸。反应应在无水条件下进行，所有试剂和反应仪器应在反应前干燥，并在反应过程中严格避水。

**安全提示**：醋酸酐和浓硫酸会引起严重烧伤。使用时应戴上手套，如果接触皮肤，立即用大量水冲洗。

## Ⅲ 实验装置和原料

### 1. 实验装置

反应实验装置如图 2-2 所示，由三颈烧瓶、球形冷凝管、磁力搅拌器和温度计等组成。
抽滤装置如图 2-3 所示，由抽滤瓶、布氏漏斗、滤纸和真空泵组成。

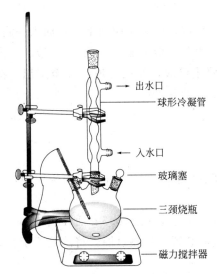

図　→ 出水口
→ 球形冷凝管
→ 入水口
→ 玻璃塞
→ 三颈烧瓶
→ 磁力搅拌器

图 2-2　反应实验装置

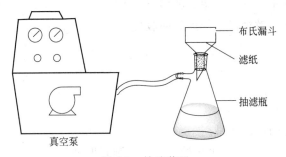

真空泵

→ 布氏漏斗
→ 滤纸
→ 抽滤瓶

图 2-3　抽滤装置

**2. 原料**

| 名称 | 用量 | 试剂级别 | 用途 |
| --- | --- | --- | --- |
| 水杨酸 | 8.3 g (0.06 mol) | 化学纯 | 反应物 |
| 醋酸酐 | 15 mL (0.159 mol) | 化学纯 | 酰化试剂 |
| 浓硫酸 | 0.4 mL (5 drops) | 化学纯 | 催化剂 |
| $FeCl_3$ 试液 | 1 滴 | — | 终点指示剂 |
| 乙醇 | 12 mL | 95% | 重结晶溶剂 |
| $H_2O$ | 适量 | — | 溶剂 |
| 活性炭 | 0.5 g | — | 脱色剂 |

# Ⅳ　实验操作

## 1. 阿司匹林粗产品的合成

（1）按图 2-2 所示搭建反应实验装置。在 100 mL 三颈烧瓶中，加入 15 mL 醋酸酐和 5 滴浓硫酸，磁搅拌状态下，升温至 55～60 ℃。

（2）在上述体系（55～60 ℃）中，加入 8.3 g 水杨酸晶体，搅拌溶解，可观察到白色晶体逐渐溶解。

（3）终点检测：取一滴反应液，滴到反应板上，再滴入一滴 $FeCl_3$ 试剂，若反应液显示淡红色，反应需要继续进行，直至反应液显示黄色（终点）。

（4）若反应达到终点，停止反应，使反应液冷却至室温，把反应瓶放入冰水浴，加入 75 mL 水，减压抽滤（图 2-3），收集产品。

（5）冰水洗涤产品 2～3 次，尽量抽干。

（6）风干粗品，称重。

**2. 阿司匹林的重结晶（纯化）**

（1）按图 2-2 所示搭建实验装置。在 100 mL 三颈烧瓶中，将阿司匹林粗品溶于 12 mL 乙醇中，升高温度至 50 ℃。

（2）待阿司匹林粗品完全溶解后，加入 0.5 g 活性炭，50 ℃下保持 5 min 以脱色。

（3）按图 2-3 搭建真空过滤装置。趁热过滤，将滤液置于实验台，冷却，加入 12 mL 冰水，再次过滤，获得阿司匹林纯品。

（4）用 30% 乙醇洗涤纯品 2～3 次，尽量抽干。

（5）风干纯品，称重，计算收率，测熔点。

（6）将产物送到指导教师指定的产品回收处。


# V  实验结果

**1. 收率**

（1）计算阿司匹林的理论产量。

$$水杨酸 ————— 阿司匹林$$
$$M_w = 138.12 \text{ g/mol} ————— M_w = 180.16 \text{ g/mol}$$
$$0.06 \text{ mol} ————— 0.06 \text{ mol}$$
$$理论产量 = 0.06 \text{ mol} \times 180.16 \text{ g/mol} = 10.81 \text{ g}$$

（2）计算阿司匹林的收率

$$收率 = \frac{产品实际产量}{产品理论产量} \times 100\% = \frac{(\quad)}{10.81 \text{ g}} \times 100\% = (\quad)\%$$

**2. 产品外观与熔点**

A. 外观：_____ ；

B. 熔点：

理论值：135～138 ℃

实测值：_____ 。

**3. 实验结果分析**

_____

_____

_____

_____

_____

## VI 注意事项

1.在阿司匹林粗品制备过程中，无水条件是至关重要的因素。这是因为醋酸酐在水中或湿空气中会发生分解，因此，该步反应需要在完全无水条件下完成。

2.在阿司匹林粗品制备过程中，反应温度控制是第二个重要的因素。这是因为浓硫酸是强氧化剂，当反应温度为 60 ℃以上时，水杨酸会被浓硫酸氧化为黄色或棕黑色产物，因此，酯化反应和重结晶温度必须控制在 60 ℃以下。

## VII 思考题

1.用结构式表示，为什么在反应过程中室内会有醋酸的味道？
2.用结构式表示，为什么水杨酸和阿司匹林是酸性物质？

（李雯　刘宏民）

# Experiment 3
# Synthesis of Paracetamol

## Background

Paracetamol（APAP），also known as acetaminophen，is a non-antiin-flammatory antipyretic analgesic drug of anilines. It has similar antipyretic effect with aspirin but weaker analgesic effect and neither anti-inflammatory nor anti-rheumatism effect.

APAP is clinically used in the treatment of fever，headache，arthralgia and neuralgia etc. Paracetamol is also the active constituent of anti-influenza compounds，such as Quike capsule for the treatment of the common cold. The chemical structure of paracetamol is shown as follow（Fig. 3-1）：

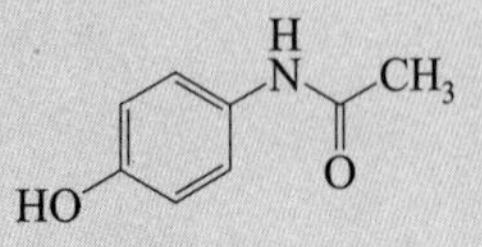

Fig. 3-1 Chemical structure of Paracetamol

APAP belongs to acetanilide drugs and its mechanism of action is still not clear but mainly through the inhibition of prostaglandin synthesis and release to achieve antipy-retic and analgesic effects. It is speculated that it exerts its effect by blocking cyclooxygenase（COX）and blocking the production of prostaglandins that mediate inflamma-tion from arachidonic acid. The inducible COX-2 enzyme is the main cyclooxygenase isoform inhibited by APAP. Here，the COX-2 protein crystal structure（PDB ID：5F1A）was selected to do docking simulation with APAP，whose ligand are the most similar to acetaminophen structure.

As can be shown from the binding mode of APAP with COX-2 and the surface map of the binding pocket（**Color Diagram 3**），a hydrogen bond formed between the acetyl carbonyloxy in paracetamol and the hydroxyl group at the side chain of Ser 530，and the benzene ring is surrounded by hydrophobic residues.

# Ⅰ  Purposes and Requirements

1. To know well and master the principle and operation techniques of acylation reaction.
2. To master the recrystallization method.
3. To know well the use of antioxidants and the protection of medicine from oxidation.
4. To understand the interaction between paracetamol and target.

# Ⅱ  Principle of the Reaction

## 1. Physical data of the main reactants and product

| Name | Structure /CAS No. | Formula / M. Wt | b. p. or m. p. /℃ | Solubility |
|---|---|---|---|---|
| p-Aminophenol | (structure) 123-30-8 | $C_6H_7NO$ 109. 13 | m. p. 188~190 | 1. 5 g/100 mL (at 20 ℃) in water, miscible with organic solvent |
| Acetic anhydride | (structure) 108-24-7 | $C_4H_6O_3$ 102. 09 | b. p. 138~139 | Reaction with water to form acetic acid and miscible with ether, chloroform and benzene |
| Paracetamol | (structure) 203-157-5 | $C_8H_9NO_2$ 151. 16 | m. p. 168~172 | 1. 4 g/100 mL (at 20 ℃) in water, miscible with organic solvent |
| Sodium hydrogen sulfite | $NaHSO_3$ 7631-90-5 | $NaHSO_3$ 104. 06 | m. p. 150~152 | Soluble in water and slightly soluble in ethanol |

## 2. Synthetic route

p-Aminophenol     Acetic anhydride          Paracetamol          Acetic acid

In this reaction, p-aminophenol will react with acetic anhydride to form paracetamol and one molecule of acetic acid.

**Safety Tips:** Acetic anhydride can cause bad burns and thus should always be used in the hood. If it comes in contact with your skin, immediately wash the area with copious amounts of water.

## Ⅲ  Experimental Equipments and Raw Materials

### 1. Experimental equipments

Acetylation reaction experimental set-up, Fig. 3-2, is composed from three-neck round-bottom flask, spherical condenser tube, constant temperature magnetic stirrer and thermometer.

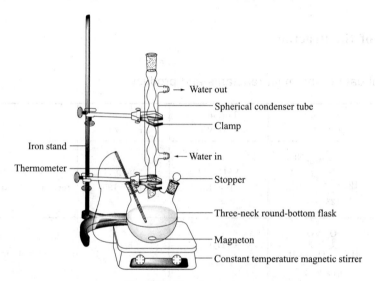

Fig. 3-2   Reaction set-up

### 2. Raw materials

| Name | Quantity | Quality | Use |
|---|---|---|---|
| $p$-Aminophenol | 10. 6 g (0. 097 mol) | C. P. | Reactant |
| Acetic anhydride | 12 mL (0. 127 mol) | C. P. | Acylation agent |
| Water | 30 mL | — | Solvent |
| Active carbon (Charcoal) | 1 g | — | Decolorization |
| $NaHSO_3$ | 0. 5 g (0. 005 mol) | C. P. | Antioxidant |

## Ⅳ  Operations

### 1. Synthesis and isolation (for obtaining the crude product)

（1）Equip the experimental set-up as shown in Fig. 3-2. Add 10. 6 g of $p$-aminophenol, 30 mL of water and 12 mL of acetic anhydride to the 100 mL three-neck round-bottom flask and agitate gently in parallel. Heat the solution to 80 ℃ on a steam bath for 30 minutes, and then cool it by putting it in ice-water bath for 20 minutes to crystallize out.

（2）Filter it and collect the crystals, wash them with 10 mL of cold water twice and dry the crystals of the obtained crude product.

## 2. Recrystallization (for purification)

(1) Equip the experimental set-up as shown in Fig. 3-2. Weigh the crude product. Place it in the 250 mL three-neck round-bottom flask and dissolve it in an adequate amount of water (the ratio is 5 mL water for 1 g of the product), and then, agitate gently in parallel. Raise the temperature to 85 ℃ to dissolve. The mixture is cooled down to 75 ℃ after dissolving. Add 1 g of active carbon to the mixture. And then, increase the temperature to 100 ℃ for boiling and keep for 5 minutes to decolor. Filter the hot reaction solution (before filter, add 0.5 g of $NaHSO_3$ into preheating filter flash to avoid oxidation of the product). The filtrate is cooled to crystallize out.

(2) Filter the mixture and collect the crystals, wash the filter cake twice with 5 mL of 0.5% $NaHSO_3$ solution.

(3) The product is dried under infrared lamp. Weigh the pure product and measure the melting point.

(4) Send the product to the place where the guide teachers designated.

# Ⅴ Experimental Results

## 1. Yield

(1) Calculate the theoretical production of paracetamol

$$p\text{-Aminophenol} \longrightarrow \text{Paracetamol}$$
$$M_w = 109.13 \text{ g/mol} \longrightarrow M_w = 151.16 \text{ g/mol}$$
$$0.097 \text{ mol} \longrightarrow 0.097 \text{ mol}$$

Theoretical production = 0.097 mol × 151.16 g/mol = 14.66 g

(2) Calculate the percent yield of paracetamol

$$\text{Yield} = \frac{\text{Practical production}}{\text{Theoretical production}} \times 100\% = \frac{(\quad)}{14.66 \text{ g}} \times 100\% = (\quad)\%$$

## 2. Appearance and melting point of product

A. Appearance: _____ ;

B. m.p. :

  Theoretical value: 169～171 ℃

  Practical value: _____ .

## 3. Analysis of experimental results

_____

_____

_____

_____

_____

_____

_____ .

# VI Notes

The purpose of adding sodium hydrogen sulfite is to avoid the oxidation of paracetamol by air. However, the concentration of sodium hydrogen sulfite should be under proper control, otherwise the product's quality will be affected.

# VII Discussion Questions

1. Can acetic acid be used as an acylating agent in this preparation?
2. What are the common acylating agents?
3. What are the common impurities of paracetamol?

(By Yajing Chen)

# 实验三
# 扑热息痛的合成

## 背景知识

扑热息痛又称对乙酰氨基酚，是一种苯胺类非抗炎解热镇痛药。它的解热作用与阿司匹林相似，镇痛作用较弱，无抗炎抗风湿作用。扑热息痛临床上常用于治疗发热、头痛、关节痛和神经痛等。扑热息痛是多种抗感冒复方制剂的活性成分，如快克胶囊。扑热息痛的化学结构式如图 3-1 所示。

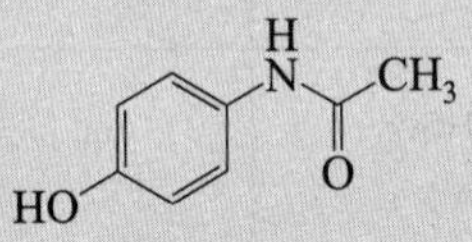

图 3-1　扑热息痛的化学结构式

对乙酰氨基酚（APAP）属于乙酰苯胺类药物，其作用机制尚不明确，主要通过抑制前列腺素的合成与释放从而达到解热、镇痛作用，分析推测其通过抑制环氧合酶（COX）而阻断花生四烯酸产生炎症介质——前列腺素，从而发挥药效作用。COX 酶中，主要由诱导型 COX-2 与发病机体相作用，选取 COX-2 蛋白晶体（PDB：5F1A，其配体与对乙酰氨基酚结构最为相似）进行分子对接。

对乙酰氨基酚在此位点的作用模式以及结合口袋的表面图如**彩插 3** 所示。其中对乙酰氨基酚中乙酰基的羰基氧与 Ser 530 侧链的羟基形成氢键，苯环与周围的氨基酸形成疏水作用。

## I　目的与要求

1. 熟悉和掌握乙酰化反应的原理和实验方法。
2. 掌握重结晶纯化方法。
3. 熟悉抗氧剂的使用及易氧化药物的保护。
4. 了解扑热息痛与靶标的作用方式。

实验三　扑热息痛的合成 | 27

## II 反应原理

### 1. 主要反应物及产物的物理常数

| 名称 | 结构式/CAS 号 | 结构式/分子量 | 熔点或沸点/℃ | 溶解度 |
|---|---|---|---|---|
| 对氨基苯酚 | 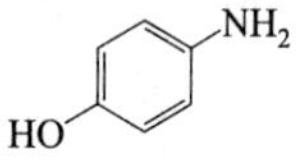 (结构式) 123-30-8 | $C_6H_7NO$ 109.13 | m. p. 188～190 | 1.5 g/100 mL（20 ℃）（水），易溶于常用有机溶剂 |
| 乙酸酐 | 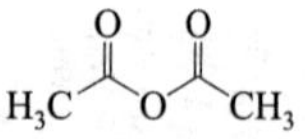 (结构式) 108-24-7 | $C_4H_6O_3$ 102.09 | b. p. 138～139 | 遇水反应，生成醋酸；易溶于乙醚，氯仿和苯 |
| 扑热息痛 | 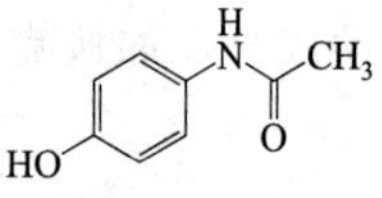 (结构式) 203-157-5 | $C_8H_9NO_2$ 151.16 | m. p. 168～172 | 1.4 g/100 mL（20 ℃）（水），易溶于常用有机溶剂 |
| 亚硫酸氢钠 | $NaHSO_3$ 7631-90-5 | $NaHSO_3$ 104.06 | m. p. 150～152 | 易溶于水，微溶于乙醇 |

### 2. 合成路线

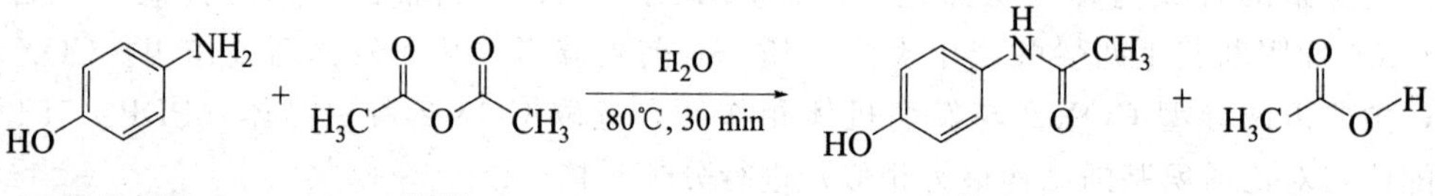

对氨基苯酚　　　　　乙酸酐　　　　　　　　　　扑热息痛　　　　　乙酸

在此反应过程中，对氨基苯酚和乙酸酐反应生成扑热息痛，同时也会产生一分子乙酸。

**安全提示**：乙酸酐可灼伤皮肤，并有刺激性味道，应在通风橱中使用。一旦接触皮肤，要立即用大量水冲洗。

## III 实验装置和原料

### 1. 实验装置

乙酰化反应实验装置如图 3-2 所示。本装置由三颈烧瓶、球形冷凝管、恒温磁力搅拌器和温度计等组成。

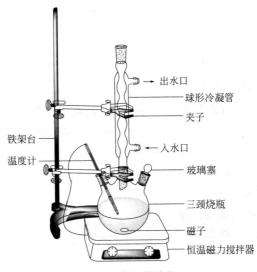

图 3-2 反应实验装置

**2. 原料**

| 名称 | 用量 | 规格 | 用途 |
|---|---|---|---|
| 对氨基苯酚 | 10.6 g (0.097 mol) | C. P. | 反应物 |
| 乙酸酐 | 12 mL (0.127 mol) | C. P. | 乙酰化试剂 |
| 水 | 30 mL | — | 溶剂 |
| 活性炭 | 1 g | — | 脱色 |
| 亚硫酸氢钠 | 0.5 g (0.005 mol) | C. P. | 抗氧剂 |

## Ⅳ 实验操作

**1. 对乙酰氨基酚的制备（粗品）**

（1）按图 3-2 所示搭建反应实验装置。于干燥的 100 mL 三颈烧瓶中加入 10.6 g 对氨基苯酚、30 mL 水和 12 mL 乙酸酐，轻轻振摇使成均相。于 80 ℃蒸汽浴中加热反应 30 min，冰水浴中冷却 20 min，析晶。

（2）抽滤，滤饼用 10 mL 冷水洗 2 次，干燥，称重。

**2. 重结晶（精制）**

（1）按图 3-2 所示搭建反应实验装置。于 250 mL 三颈烧瓶中，加入对乙酰氨基酚粗品，每克粗品用水 5 mL，加入计算量的水作溶剂，加热至 85 ℃使其溶解，溶解后稍冷至 75 ℃，加入 1 g 活性炭，重新加热至 100 ℃，煮沸 5 min。

（2）趁热抽滤（抽滤前，将布氏漏斗和抽滤瓶在 80 ℃烘箱中预热 30 min，并在预热后的抽滤瓶中先加入 0.5 g 亚硫酸氢钠），滤液冷却析晶。滤饼以 0.5% 亚硫酸氢钠溶液 5 mL 分 2 次洗涤，抽滤，干燥，得白色的对乙酰氨基酚纯品。

（3）烘干纯品，称重，计算收率，测熔点。

（4）将产物送到指导教师指定的产品回收处。

## V 实验结果

### 1. 收率

（1）计算扑热息痛的理论产量

$$对氨基苯酚 \text{————} 对乙酰氨基酚$$
$$M_w = 109.13 \text{ g/mol} \text{————} M_w = 151.16 \text{ g/mol}$$
$$0.097 \text{ mol} \text{————} 0.097 \text{ mol}$$
$$理论产量 = 0.097 \text{ mol} \times 151.16 \text{ g/mol} = 14.66 \text{ g}$$

（2）计算扑热息痛的收率

$$收率 = \frac{产品实际产量}{产品理论产量} \times 100\% = \frac{(\quad)}{14.66 \text{ g}} \times 100\% = (\quad)\%$$

### 2. 产品外观与熔点

A. 外观：_____；

B. 熔点：

  理论值：169～171 ℃

  实测值：_____。

### 3. 实验结果分析

_____

_____

_____

_____

_____

_____

_____

_____。

## VI 注意事项

加亚硫酸氢钠可防止对乙酰氨基酚被空气氧化，但亚硫酸氢钠浓度不宜过高，否则会影响产品质量。

## VII 思考题

1. 本实验中乙酸可以作为乙酰化试剂来使用吗？

2. 常用的乙酰化试剂有哪些？

3. 合成扑热息痛时常见的杂质有哪些？

（陈亚静）

# Experiment 4
# Synthesis of Benorilate

## Background

Benorilate is a prodrug formed by the combination of aspirin and paracetamol. Clinically, it is used for the treatment of rheumatoid arthritis, cold-fervescence, neuralgia and others. The curative effect of benorilate is similar to that of aspirin, but with longer duration of action and fewer side effects. The chemical structure of benorilate is shown as follow Fig. 4-1.

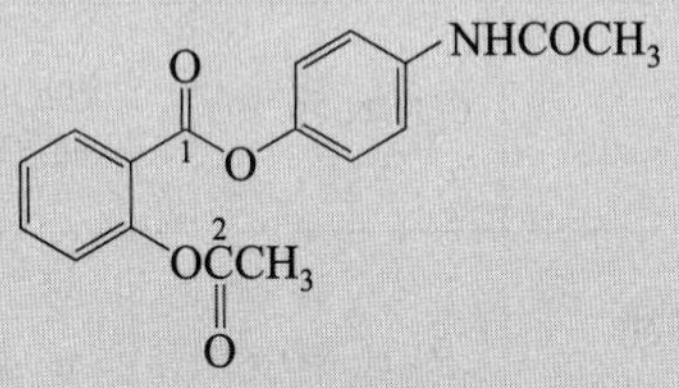

Fig. 4-1.   Chemical structure of Benorilate

The mechanism of benorilate is basically similar to that of aspirin and acetaminophen. The complex crystal structure of the cyclooxygenase COX-2 and benorilate (PDB: 5F1A) are used to determine the binding mode. As shown in **Color Diagram 4**, there is a hydrogen bond formed between the ester carbonyl oxygen at the 1-position of benorilate and the hydroxyl group at the side chain of Ser 530. The carbonyl oxygen at the acetyloxy group at the 2-position also forms a hydrogen bond with the hydroxyl group at the side chain of Tyr 385. In addition, the benzene ring forms hydrophobic interactions with the surrounding hydrophobic residues.

## I  Purposes and Requirements

1. To understand the principle of chlorization reaction and its requirements.

2. To understand the application of combination principle in chemical structure modification.

3. To learn the treatment method of toxic gas produced during the reaction.

4. To master the technique of anhydrous operation of the reaction.

5. To understand the principle of Schotten-Baumann esterification.

6. To understand the interaction between benorilate and target.

## II Principle of the Reaction

### 1. Physical data of the main reactants and product

| Name | Structure /CAS No. | Formula / M. Wt | b. p. or m. p. /℃ | Solubility |
|---|---|---|---|---|
| Aspirin | COOH / OCOCH$_3$ / 50-78-2 | C$_9$H$_8$O$_4$ 180.16 | m. p. 135~138 | In water: 3.3 g/L (at 20 ℃) In DMSO: 100 mmol/L (at 20 ℃) |
| 2-(Acetyloxy)-benzoylchlorid | COCl / OCOCH$_3$ / 5538-51-2 | C$_9$H$_7$O$_3$Cl 198.60 | m. p. 45~49 | Soluble in toluene Decomposed in water |
| Thionyl chloride | SOCl$_2$ 7719-09-7 | SOCl$_2$ 118.96 | b. p. 79 | React with water and miscible with organic solvents |
| Pyridine | N / 110-86-1 | C$_5$H$_5$N 79.10 | m. p. 96~98 | Soluble in water and common organic solvents |
| Paracetamol | H N CH$_3$ / HO O / 203-157-5 | C$_8$H$_9$NO$_2$ 151.16 | m. p. 168~172 | In water: 1.4 g/100 mL (at 20 ℃) Miscible in organic solvent In ethanol: 0.5 mol/L (at 20 ℃) |
| Benorilate | O NHCOCH$_3$ / OCOCH$_3$ / 5003-48-5 | C$_{17}$H$_{15}$NO$_5$ 313.31 | m. p. 177~181 | Insoluble in water Easily soluble in hot ethanol |

### 2. Synthetic route

(1) 
$$\begin{array}{c}\text{COOH}\\\text{OCOCH}_3\end{array} + SOCl_2 \xrightarrow{\text{N}} \begin{array}{c}\text{COCl}\\\text{OCOCH}_3\end{array} + HCl + SO_2$$

(2)
$$\begin{array}{c}\text{H}\\\text{N}\quad\text{CH}_3\\\text{HO}\quad\text{O}\end{array} + NaOH \longrightarrow \begin{array}{c}\text{H}\\\text{N}\quad\text{CH}_3\\\text{NaO}\quad\text{O}\end{array} + H_2O$$

(3)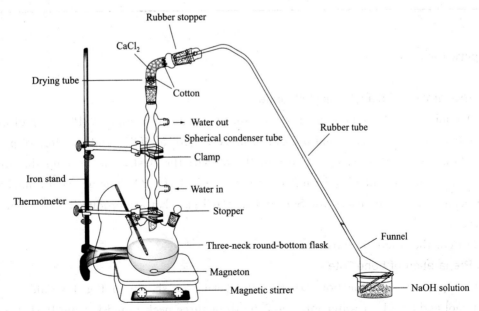

During Benorilate synthesis, the phenol group of paracetamol reacts with the carboxyl group of aspirin to form an ester product. Aspirin is an aromatic acid which has low reactivity. In this experiment, aspirin is first treated with thionyl chloride and pyridine to forming the corresponding acetyl salicylic chloride under anhydrous reaction condition. Considering the similar low reactivity of phenol group of the paracetamol, paracetamol is changed to its sodium salt in sodium hydroxide solution. Finally, the two intermediates formed then react at room temperature to form benorilate.

**Safety Tips:** Thionyl chloride and pyridine have irritating smell and thus should be used in the fume hood. They can burn the skin and irritate the mucous membrane. Thionyl chloride and the produced acetyl salicylic chloride can react violently with water and liberate toxic gas.

## Ⅲ Experimental Equipments and Raw Materials

### 1. Experimental equipments

Chlorization experimental set-up, Fig. 4-2, is composed from magnetic stirrer, three-neck round-bottom flask, spherical condenser tube, thermometer, drying tube containing calcium chloride, gas-guide tube, funnel and NaOH absorption solution.

Fig. 4-2 Chlorization experimental set-up

Esterification experimental set-up, Fig. 4-3, is composed from magnetic stirrer, ice-water bath, three-neck round-bottom flask, thermometer and constant pressure funnel.

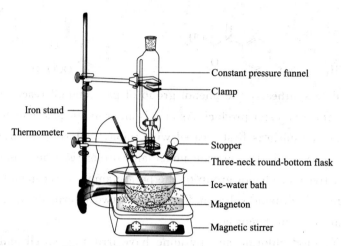

Constant pressure funnel
Clamp

Iron stand

Thermometer

Stopper
Three-neck round-bottom flask
Ice-water bath
Magneton
Magnetic stirrer

Fig. 4-3   Esterification experimental set-up

## 2. Raw materials

| Name | Quantity | Quality | Use |
| --- | --- | --- | --- |
| Aspirin | 9 g (0. 05 mol) | Officinal | Reactant |
| Thionyl chloride | 5 mL (0. 069 mol) | C. P. | Chlorization reagent |
| Pyridine | 1 drop | C. P. | Catalyst |
| Paracetamol | 8. 6 g (0. 57 mol) | Officinal | Reactant |
| Sodium hydroxide | 3. 3 g (0. 083 mol) | C. P. | Base |
| Anhydrous acetone | 6 mL | A. R. | Solvent |
| Water | 50 mL | — | Solvent |

# Ⅳ  Operations

## 1. Preparation of acetyl salicyl chloride

(1) Equip the chlorization experimental set-up as shown in Fig. 4-2. Place 9 g of aspirin in the 100 mL of three-neck round-bottom flask. Add 5 mL of $SOCl_2$ and one drop of pyridine in the 100 mL of three-neck round-bottom flask. Swirl the flask, and heat up the mixture slowly to 75 ℃ and maintain the temperature at 70~75 ℃ for 2 h. The inverted funnel in the beaker serves as trap to absorb the $SO_2$ and the HCl gas that are produced during the reaction process.

(2) Cool the reaction mixture and keep it.

## 2. Preparation of benorilate

(1) Equip the esterification experimental set-up as shown in Fig. 4-3. Add 8. 6 g of paracetamol and 50 mL of water into the 250 mL of three-neck round-bottom flask. Cool the reaction mixture in an ice-water bath to 10~15 ℃. Add sodium hydroxide solution (3. 3 g NaOH in 18 mL of $H_2O$) with a dropper and keep the temperature at 10~15 ℃. Cool the reaction mixture to 8~12 ℃.

(2) Add 3 mL of anhydrous acetone to the above acyl chloride mixture and transfer the solution to a dry constant pressure funnel. Repeat the operation once more. Under strong agitation, add the acetonic solution of acetyl salicyl chloride dropwise by the constant pressure drop funnel to the above reaction mixture. Regulate the pH value to 9~10. Remove the ice-water bath and keep the reaction temperature at 20~25 ℃ for 2 h.

(3) Filter the mixture by suction and wash it by cold water until the pH becomes neutral for obtaining the crude product Benorilate.

(4) Dry the product under infrared lamp. Weigh the pure product and measure the melting point.

(5) Send the finished product to the place where the guide teachers designated.

## V Experimental Results

### 1. Yield
(1) Calculate the theoretical production of benorilate

$$\text{Aspirin} \longrightarrow \text{Benorilate}$$
$$M_w = 180.16 \text{ g/mol} \longrightarrow M_w = 313.3 \text{ g/mol}$$
$$0.05 \text{ mol} \longrightarrow 0.05 \text{ mol}$$
$$\text{Theoretical production} = 0.05 \text{ mol} \times 313.3 \text{ g/mol} = 15.67 \text{ g}$$

(2) Calculate the percent yield of benorilate

$$\text{Yield} = \frac{\text{Practical production}}{\text{Theoretical production}} \times 100\% = \frac{(\quad)}{15.67 \text{ g}} \times 100\% = (\quad)\%$$

### 2. Appearance and melting point of product
A. Appearance: _____ ;

B. m. p. :

   Theoretical value: 175~176 ℃

   Practical value: _____ .

### 3. Analysis of experimental results

_____

_____

_____

_____

_____

_____

_____ .

## VI Notes

1. The reaction of chlorization (the first reaction) should take place under dry condition (All the apparatus and reagents mustn't contain water fraction). For this, the glass appara-

tus will be dried and a drying tube which contains calcium chloride should be placed on the top of the condenser.

2. It is necessary to install the toxic gas treating apparatus, to avoid the harmful effect of toxic gas produced during the reaction.

3. Reaction mixture must be slowly heated to prevent the formation of the by-products.

4. The amount of pyridine used as a catalyst should not be excessive, otherwise the quality of the product will be affected.

5. The temperature must be controlled strictly at 70~75 ℃, and should not exceed 80 ℃. Too low temperature isn't beneficial to the reaction while thionyl chloride will be volatile when the temperature is too high.

## Ⅶ Discussion Questions

1. Why benorilate cannot be prepared directly from aspirin and paracetamol?

2. What are the common reagents for the preparation of carboxylic chloride from carboxylic acid?

3. Why should some pyridine be added in the preparation of acetyl salicylic chloride? What will happen if pyridine is added in excess?

(By Yajing Chen)

# 实验四

# 苯乐来的合成

## 背景知识

苯乐来（Benorilate），又名扑炎痛、贝诺酯、百乐来，是一种解热镇痛药。苯乐来是一种前药，由阿司匹林和扑热息痛缩合而成。在临床上，常用于治疗风湿性关节炎、感冒发热和神经痛等。苯乐来的疗效和阿司匹林相似，却有更长的作用时间及较少的副作用。苯乐来化学结构如图 4-1 所示。

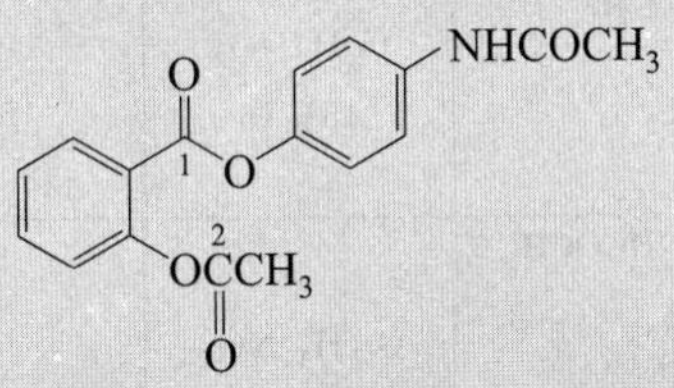

图 4-1　苯乐来的化学结构式

苯乐来作用于环氧合酶-2（COX-2），采用与阿司匹林结合最好的晶体蛋白（PDB：5F1A）与苯乐来进行对接实验。如**彩插 4A** 所示，COX-2 与水杨酸的复合晶体结构（PDB：5F1A）及其活性位点，可以用于确定苯乐来的结合位点。分子模拟结果显示苯乐来可以与水杨酸结合位点形成良好的相互作用（**彩插 4B**）。苯乐来在此位点的作用模式以及结合口袋的表面图如**彩插 4** 所示。其中苯乐来中 1 位酯羰基氧与 Ser 530 侧链的羟基形成氢键，2 位上乙酰氧基上的羰基氧与 Tyr 385 侧链的羟基形成氢键，苯环与周围的氨基酸形成疏水作用。

## I　目的与要求

1. 理解制备酰氯化合物的反应原理及操作。
2. 理解拼合原理在化学结构修饰方面的应用。
3. 学习反应过程中产生的有毒气体的处理方法。
4. 掌握无水操作的方法。
5. 理解 Schotten-Baumann 酯化反应的原理。
6. 了解苯乐来与靶标的作用方式。

## II 反应原理

### 1. 主要反应物和产物的物理常数

| 名称 | 结构式<br>/CAS 号 | 分子式<br>/分子量 | 熔点或<br>沸点/℃ | 溶解度 |
|---|---|---|---|---|
| 阿司匹林 | COOH OCOCH$_3$<br>50-78-2 | C$_9$H$_8$O$_4$<br>180.16 | m. p.<br>135~138 | 20 ℃ 水中溶解度为<br>3.3 g/L,20 ℃ DMSO 中溶<br>解度 100 mmol/L |
| 邻乙酰水杨酰氯 | COCl OCOCH$_3$<br>5538-51-2 | C$_9$H$_7$O$_3$Cl<br>198.16 | m. p.<br>45~49 | 溶于甲苯,遇水分解 |
| 二氯亚砜 | SOCl$_2$<br>7719-09-7 | SOCl$_2$<br>118.97 | b. p.<br>79 | 和水反应;可溶于常用<br>有机溶剂 |
| 吡啶 | N<br>110-86-1 | C$_5$H$_5$N<br>79.1 | b. p.<br>96~98 | 可溶于水和常用有机溶<br>剂 |
| 扑热息痛 | H N CH$_3$ HO O<br>203-157-5 | C$_8$H$_9$NO$_2$<br>151.16 | m. p.<br>168~172 | 20 ℃ 水中溶解度为<br>14 g/L,20 ℃ 乙醇中溶解<br>度为 500 mmol/L,与有机<br>溶剂混溶 |
| 苯乐来 | O NHCOCH$_3$ O OCOCH$_3$<br>5003-48-5 | C$_17$H$_15$NO$_5$<br>313.3 | m. p.<br>177~181 | 不溶于水<br>易溶于热的乙醇 |

### 2. 合成路线

(1) COOH OCOCH$_3$ + SOCl$_2$ $\xrightarrow{\text{N}}$ COCl OCOCH$_3$ + HCl + SO$_2$

(2) H N CH$_3$ HO O + NaOH $\longrightarrow$ H N CH$_3$ NaO O + H$_2$O

(3) COCl OCOCH$_3$ + H N CH$_3$ NaO O $\longrightarrow$ O NHCOCH$_3$ O OCOCH$_3$ + NaCl

  苯乐来是由阿司匹林和扑热息痛缩合而成,即扑热息痛的羟基和阿司匹林羧基发生酯化反应。在本实验中,低活性的阿司匹林首先在吡啶的催化作用下和氯化亚砜反应生成高活性的乙酰水杨酰氯;同样的,低活性的扑热息痛在碱性作用下生成高活性的钠盐,然后,高活性的乙酰水杨酰氯和扑热息痛钠盐在室温下生成苯乐来。

**安全提示**：氯化亚砜和吡啶有刺激性气味，必须在通风橱中使用，它们能灼伤皮肤，刺激黏膜。氯化亚砜及酰氯遇水剧烈反应，并且产生有毒气体。

## Ⅲ 实验装置和原料

### 1. 实验装置

氯化实验装置参见图 4-2。该装置由磁力搅拌器、三颈烧瓶、球形冷凝管、温度计、干燥管、导气管、漏斗和 NaOH 吸收液等组成。

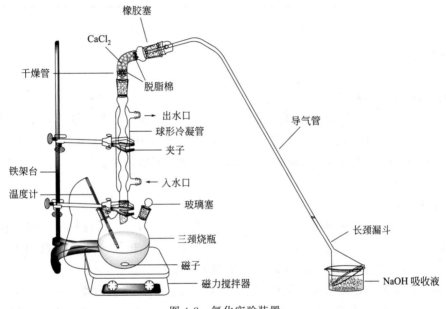

图 4-2　氯化实验装置

酯化实验装置参见图 4-3。该装置由磁力搅拌器、冰水浴、三颈烧瓶、温度计和恒压滴液漏斗等组成。

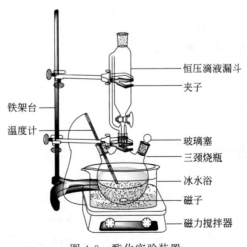

图 4-3　酯化实验装置

**2. 原料**

| 名称 | 用量 | 规格 | 用途 |
|------|------|------|------|
| 阿司匹林 | 9 g（0.05 mol） | 药用 | 反应物 |
| 氯化亚砜 | 5 mL（0.069 mol） | 化学纯 | 氯化试剂 |
| 吡啶 | 1 滴 | 化学纯 | 催化剂 |
| 扑热息痛 | 8.6 g（0.57 mol） | 药用 | 反应物 |
| 氢氧化钠 | 3.3 g（0.083 mol） | 化学纯 | 碱 |
| 无水丙酮 | 6 mL | 分析纯 | 溶剂 |
| 水 | 50 mL | — | 溶剂 |

## Ⅳ 实验操作

**1. 乙酰水杨酰氯的制备**

（1）按图 4-2 所示搭建氯化实验装置。于干燥的 100 mL 三颈烧瓶中，加入阿司匹林 9 g、氯化亚砜 5 mL 及 1 滴吡啶。缓缓加热至 75 ℃，维持 70～75 ℃，保温反应 2 h。将生成的 $SO_2$ 和 HCl 有害气体通过长颈漏斗导入到氢氧化钠吸收液中。

（2）冷却，密封备用。

**2. 苯乐来的制备**

（1）按图 4-3 所示搭建酯化实验装置。于干燥的 250 mL 三颈烧瓶中，加入扑热息痛 8.6 g 和水 50 mL。冰水浴中冷却混合物温度至 10～15 ℃。于 10～15 ℃缓缓加入氢氧化钠液 18 mL（3.3 g NaOH 加水至 18 mL）。降温至 8～12 ℃。

（2）在上述制备的乙酰水杨酰氯中加入 3 mL 无水丙酮并将该丙酮溶液转移至干燥的恒压滴液漏斗中，再次向乙酰水杨酰氯储存瓶中加入 3 mL 无水丙酮并将该溶液一并转移至恒压滴液漏斗中。缓慢滴加上述制备的 6 mL 乙酰水杨酰氯无水丙酮液。调节 pH 至 9～10，撤去冰水浴，于 20～25 ℃搅拌反应 2 h。

（3）反应完毕，抽滤，用水洗至中性，得产品。

（4）烘干纯品，称重，计算收率，测熔点。

（5）将产物送到指导教师指定的产品回收处。

## Ⅴ 实验结果

**1. 收率**

（1）计算苯乐来的理论产量

$$阿司匹林————苯乐来$$
$$M_w=180.16 \text{ g/mol} ————M_w=313.3 \text{ g/mol}$$
$$0.05 \text{ mol} ————0.05 \text{ mol}$$
$$理论产量=0.05 \text{ mol}×313.3 \text{ g/mol}=15.67 \text{ g}$$

（2）计算苯乐来的收率

$$收率 = \frac{产品实际产量}{产品理论产量} \times 100\% = \frac{(\quad)}{15.67\ g} \times 100\% = (\quad)\%$$

**2. 产品外观与熔点**

A. 外观： _____ ；

B. 熔点：

    理论值：175～176 ℃

    实测值： _____ 。

**3. 实验结果分析**

_____

_____

_____

_____

_____

_____

_____

_____ 。

## VI 注意事项

1. 第一步氯化反应需在无水条件下操作，因此，实验前，需要将所有玻璃仪器都干燥，回流冷凝管顶部需加一个氯化钙干燥管。

2. 因为反应会生成氯化氢和二氧化硫有毒气体，因此需要使用尾气吸收装置。

3. 为了避免副产物的生成，反应要缓慢升温。

4. 吡啶不可过量，否则影响产品的质量和产量。

5. 反应过程中，注意控制温度在 70～75 ℃ 为佳。若反应温度过低，不利于反应进行；温度太高，氯化亚砜易挥发。

## VII 思考题

1. 为何不直接用阿司匹林和扑热息痛制备苯乐来？

2. 由羧酸制备酰氯的常用方法有哪些？

3. 由羧酸和氯化亚砜制备酰氯时，为什么要加入少量吡啶？吡啶的量若加多了会发生什么后果？

（陈亚静）

# Experiment 5

# Synthesis of Sulfacetamide Sodium

## Background

The sulfanilamides derivatives of *p*-aminobenzene sulfonamide parent ring (Fig. 5-1), the earliest synthetic antibacterial drugs, play an important role in the treatment of infectious diseases with broad antibacterial spectrum, oral and rapid absorption. Bacteria can not directly utilize folic acid in the environment, but synthesis dihydrofolic acid by *p*-aminobenzoic acid (PABA) with dihydropteroate synthase (DHPS) which is a key enzyme in the folate pathway of bacteria (Fig. 5-1). In a reaction catalyzed by dihydrofolate reductase dihydrofolic acid is converted to tetrahydrofolic acid which is used for the synthesis of nucleic acid precurssors such as purines, and hence essential for bacterial growth and proliferation. In this experiment, sulfacetamide sodium which is a short-acting sulfonamide and a structural analog of PABA is synthesized (Fig. 5-1).

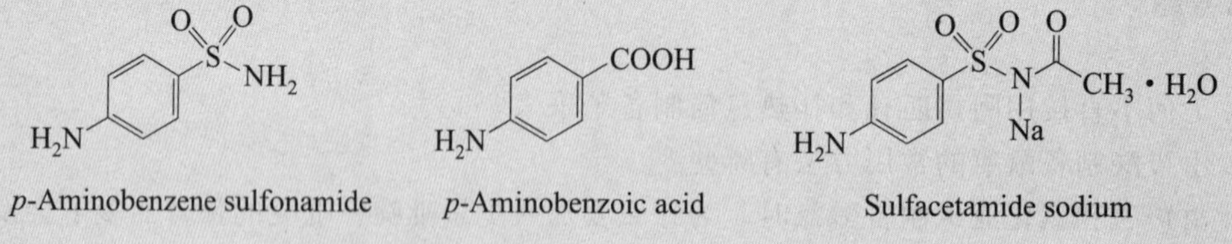

*p*-Aminobenzene sulfonamide     *p*-Aminobenzoic acid     Sulfacetamide sodium

Fig. 5-1　The structure of *p*-Aminobenzene sulfonamide, *p*-Aminobenzoic acid and Sulfacetamide sodium

Studies have shown that sulfonamides can compete with *p*-aminobenzoic acid for bacterial dihydrofolate synthase, which hinders the metabolism of bacteria, prevents the acquisition of purine and nucleic acid required, and inhibits the growth and reproduction of bacteria. The co-crystal structure of

PABA with dihydropteroate synthase (PDB: 3TYZ) directly shows the active site of PABA. Then, molecular docking, a molecular modeling method, predicts that sulfacetamide sodium can bind with the active site well (MOE software). Furthermore, sulfacetamide sodium competes with PABA to prevent bacterial folic acid synthesis. The predicted binding mode and surface of the active site are shown in **Color Diagram 5.**

## I  Purposes and Requirements

1. To understand the general physical and chemical properties of sulfanilamides, and to know how to purify the product by using these properties.

2. To master the principle and the operation of acetylation.

3. To understand the interaction between sulfacetamide sodium and target.

## II  Principle of the Reaction

### 1. Physical data of the main reactants and product

| Name | Structure /CAS No. | Formula / M. Wt | b. p. or m. p. /℃ | Solubility |
|---|---|---|---|---|
| Sulfanilamide | H$_2$N—⟨⟩—SO$_2$NH$_2$<br>63-74-1 | $C_6H_8N_2O_2S$<br>172. 21 | m. p.<br>165~166 | Slightly soluble in cold water and ethanol; soluble in NaOH solution; Insoluble in chloroform, ether |
| Sulfacetamide | H$_2$N—⟨⟩—SO$_2$NHCOCH$_3$<br>144-80-9 | $C_8H_{10}N_2SO_3$<br>214. 24 | m. p.<br>179~184 | Soluble in ethanol, slightly soluble in water or ether |
| Sulfacetamide Sodium | H$_2$N—⟨⟩—S(=O)(=O)—N(Na)—C(=O)CH$_3$ · H$_2$O<br>127-56-0 | $C_8H_9N_2NaO_3S \cdot H_2O$<br>254. 24 | m. p.<br>183 | Soluble in water, slightly soluble in ethanol and acetone |
| Acetic anhydride | H$_3$C—C(=O)—O—C(=O)—CH$_3$<br>108-24-7 | $C_4H_6O_3$<br>102. 09 | b. p.<br>138~139 | Reaction with water to form acetic acid and miscible with ether, chloroform and benzene |

## 2. Synthetic route

In this reaction, synthesis of sulfacetamide sodium is by the way that sulfacetamide is prepared by acetylation of sulfanilamide. Sulfacetamide is then reacts with sodium hydroxide aqueous solution in ethanol to generate its sodium salt. There are two amino groups in the structure of sulfanilamide and diacetylated products can be produced. In this acetylation process the issue of specificity should be considered. The pH of the reaction is very important and the key to control the specificity of the synthesis route as well as the separation and crystallization of the final reaction product.

The dissolution of the products and by-products at different pH are shown in Table 5-1. The dissolution and precipitation of the products and by-products during the experiment are shown in Fig. 5-2. During the operation, attention should be paid to distinguishing the filtrate from the filter cake.

Table 5-1　The dissolution of the products and by-products at different pH

| Name | pH＝7 | pH＝4～5 | pH＜2 |
|---|---|---|---|
| Sulfanilamide | Very low solubility | Dissolve | Dissolve |
| Sulfacetamide | Dissolve | Low solubility | Dissolve |
| Diacetylation products | Dissolve | Low solubility | Insoluble |

**Safety Tips:** Like other corrosive acids and alkalis, drops of sodium hydroxide solutions can readily cause chemical burns and may induce permanent blindness upon contact with eyes. Thus, protective equipment, like rubber gloves, safety tips clothing and eye protection, should always be used when handling this chemical or its solutions. The standard first aid measure for alkali spills on the skin is, as for other corrosives, irrigation with large quantities of water. Washing is continued for at least fifteen minutes.

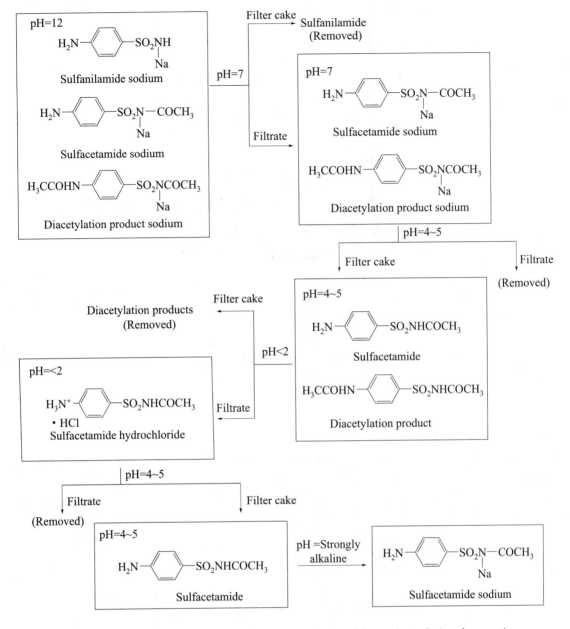

Fig. 5-2　The dissolution and precipitation of the products and by-products during the experiment

## Ⅲ Experimental Equipments and Raw Materials

### 1. Experimental equipments

Reflux experimental set-up, Fig. 5-3, is composed from three-neck round-bottom flask, spherical condenser tube, magnetic stirrer and thermometer.

Basification experimental set-up, Fig. 5-4, is composed from constant temperature magnetic stirrer and breaker.

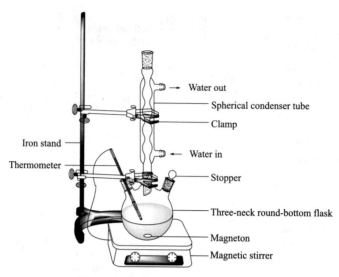

Fig. 5-3 Reflux experimental set-up

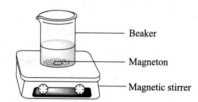

Fig. 5-4 Basification experimental set-up

## 2. Raw materials

| Materials | Quantity | Quality | Use |
|---|---|---|---|
| Sulfanilamide | 17. 2 g (0. 1 mol) | C. P. | Material |
| Acetic anhydride | 13. 6 mL (0. 14 mol) | C. P. | Acetylating agent |
| Sodium hydroxide | 22 mL (0. 11 mol) | 22. 5% | Material |
| | 12. 5 mL (0. 19 mol) | 77% | Material |
| | Proper amount | 40% | Adjusting pH |
| Concentrated hydrochloric acid | Proper amount | — | Adjusting pH |
| Diluted hydrochloric acid | Proper amount | 10% | Solvent |
| Active carbon (Charcoal) | 0. 5 g | — | Decolorization |
| Sodium hydroxide-ethanol | Proper amount | 5% | Generating sodium salt |
| Water | Proper amount | — | Dilution |

## Ⅳ Operations

### 1. The preparation of sulfacetamide

（1）Equip the reflux experimental set-up as shown in Fig. 5-3. Add Sulfanilamide 17. 2 g and 22.5% sodium hydroxide aqueous solution 22 mL into the 100 mL three-necked round-bottom flask. Then stir the mixture and heated to 50 ℃.

(2) After the mixture is completely dissolved, add acetic anhydride 3.6 mL drop-wise. And 5 minutes later, add 2.5 mL sodium hydroxide aqueous solution (77%) and the pH of the reaction solution should be kept between 12 and 13. Then add acetic anhydride and sodium hydroxide aqueous solutions dropwise every 5 minutes alternately in an alternative manner (2 mL each time). During the addition of materials, the reaction temperature should be maintained at 50～55 ℃ and the pH between 12 and 13.

(3) After that, maintain the reaction mixture at 50～55 ℃ for 30 minutes with stirring.

(4) Pour the reaction mixture into a 100 mL beaker and dilute it with 20 mL water. Adjust the pH is to 7 with concentrated hydrochloric acid. Then put in ice-water bath for 20～30 minutes in order to precipitate the solid.

(5) Collect the solid by suction and wash with proper amount of ice water. Then combine the above filtered solution and washed solution, adjust the pH to 4～5 with concentrated hydrochloric acid. Collect the solid and dry it by suction.

(6) Dissolve the precipitate with 10% hydrochloric acid (3 times the volume of the precipitate). Let the solution settled for 30 minutes and remove the undissolved solid by filtration. Next, add 1 g of activated charcoal to the filtrate to decolorize at room temperature. After suction filtration, adjust the pH of the filtrate (pH=5) with 40% sodium hydroxide solution. Sulfacetamide precipitates from the solution and is collected by suction.

(7) Dry the product under infrared lamp. Weigh the pure product and measure the melting point. If the melting point is unqualified, it is refined with hot water (1 ∶ 15).

### 2. The preparation of sodium sulfacetamide

(1) Equip the basification experimental set-up as shown in Fig. 5-4. Put the above obtained sulfacetamide into the 100 mL beaker. Add 5% sodium hydroxide ethanol solution (4 times volume of the product), stir it at room temperature until the solid is completely dissolved and then precipitat out the solid product from the solution. Collect the solid by suction and washed it with an proper amount of ethanol.

(2) Dry the product under infrared lamp. Weigh the pure product and measure the melting point.

(3) Send the final product to the place where the guide teachers designated.

# Ⅴ  Experimental Results

### 1. Yield

(1) Calculate the theoretical production of sulfacetamide sodium

$$\text{Sulfanilamide} \longrightarrow \text{Sulfacetamide Sodium}$$
$$M_w = 172.21 \text{ g/mol} \longrightarrow M_w = 254.24 \text{ g/mol}$$
$$0.1 \text{ mol} \longrightarrow 0.1 \text{ mol}$$
$$\text{Theoretical production} = 0.1 \text{ mol} \times 254.24 \text{ g/mol} = 25.42 \text{ g}$$

(2) Calculate the percent yield of sulfacetamide sodium

$$\text{Yield} = \frac{\text{Practical production}}{\text{Theoretical production}} \times 100\% = \frac{(\quad)}{25.42\ \text{g}} \times 100\% = (\quad)\%$$

2. Appearance and melting point of product

A. Appearance: _____ ;

B. m. p. :

    Theoretical value: 179~184 ℃

    Practical value: _____ .

3. Analysis of experimental results

_____

_____

_____

_____

_____

_____

_____ .

## Ⅵ  Notes

1. In these experiment, different concentrations of sodium hydroxide aqueous solution are used. Careful operation is necessary.

2. Acetic anhydride and sodium hydroxide aqueous solution should be added every five minutes. After adding one of these solutions, allow it to react for 5 minutes, and then adding another solution. The solution should be added drop by drop.

3. It is important to keep the pH of the solution between 12 and 13 during the reaction, otherwise the yield will be reduced.

4. Precipitate different solid product under different pH conditions. Don't get confused.

## Ⅶ  Discussion Questions

1. During the reaction, what are the solids precipitated at pH=7 and pH=5? What is the insoluble solid in 10% hydrochloric acid?

2. During the reaction, it is very important to adjust pH between 12 and 13, and what will happen if alkaline is too strong or too weak?

(By Lina Ding)

## 背景知识

具有对氨基苯磺酰胺结构片段（图 5-1）的磺胺类药物是应用最早的一类化学合成抗菌药，在治疗感染性疾病中起着重要作用，具有抗菌谱广、可以口服、吸收较迅速等特点。

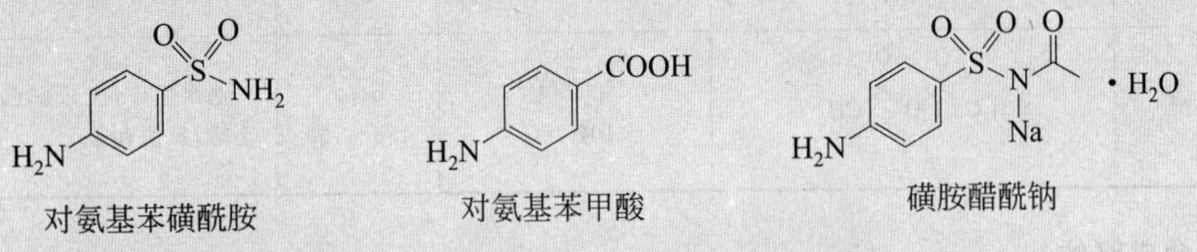

图 5-1　对氨基苯磺酰胺、对氨基苯甲酸及磺胺醋酰钠的结构式

一般情况下，细菌不能直接利用环境中的叶酸，而是通过二氢叶酸合成酶将环境中的对氨基苯甲酸（$p$-Aminobenzoic acid，PABA）催化合成二氢叶酸，进一步生成核酸前体（嘌呤、嘧啶）。核酸是细菌生长繁殖的必需成分。大量研究表明，磺胺类药物能与对氨基苯甲酸竞争细菌的二氢叶酸合成酶，使细菌的代谢受阻，无法获得生长繁殖所需的嘌呤和核酸，从而致使细菌生长繁殖受到抑制。本实验中所涉及的磺胺醋酰钠是短效磺胺类药物，如图 5-1 所示，其结构与对氨基苯甲酸结构类似。二氢叶酸合成酶（PDB：3TYZ）与对氨基苯甲酸的复合晶体结构可以清楚显示对氨基苯甲酸的结合位点，通过分子对接模拟，采用 MOE 软件预测磺胺醋酰钠可以很好地结合在该活性位点，与环境中对氨基苯甲酸竞争性结合活性位点，从而发挥抗菌作用。模拟预测的结合模式以及结合位点的表面图如彩插 5 所示。

## Ⅰ　目的与要求

1. 通过本实验，掌握磺胺类药物的一般理化性质，并掌握如何利用其理化性质的特点来达到分离提纯产品的目的。

2. 通过本实验操作，掌握乙酰化反应的原理。

3. 了解磺胺醋酰钠与靶标的作用方式。

## Ⅱ 实验原理

### 1. 主要反应物、产物的物理性质

| 试剂名称 | 结构式/CAS号 | 分子式/分子量 | 沸点或熔点/℃ | 溶解度 |
|---|---|---|---|---|
| 磺胺 | 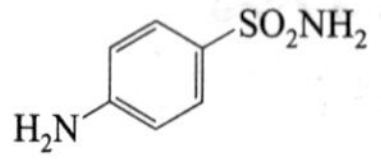 （结构式）63-74-1 | $C_6H_8N_2O_2S$ 172.21 | m. p. 165~166 | 微溶于冷水、乙醇,易溶于NaOH溶液,不溶于氯仿、乙醚 |
| 磺胺醋酰 | 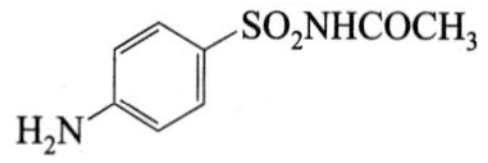 （结构式）144-80-9 | $C_8H_{10}N_2SO_3$ 214.24 | m. p. 179~184 | 溶于乙醇,微溶于水或乙醚 |
| 磺胺醋酰钠 | 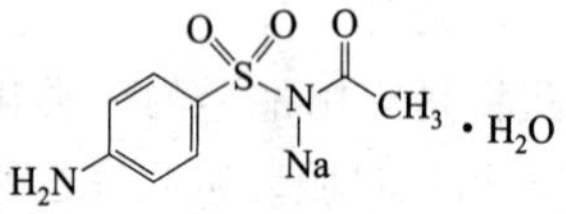 （结构式）127-56-0 | $C_8H_9N_2NaO_3S \cdot H_2O$ 254.24 | m. p. 183 | 易溶于水,微溶于乙醇、丙酮 |
| 醋酸酐 | 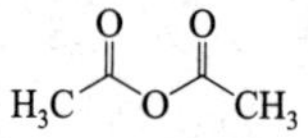 （结构式）108-24-7 | $C_4H_6O_3$ 102.09 | b. p. 138~139 | 遇水反应,生成醋酸;易溶于乙醚、氯仿和苯 |

### 2. 合成路线

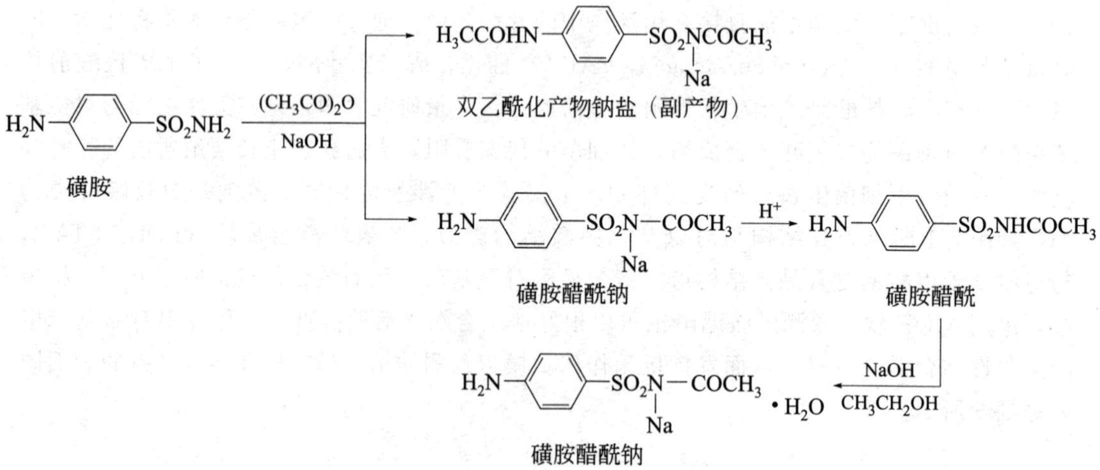

磺胺醋酰钠的合成首先通过磺胺的乙酰化制备磺胺醋酰,而后在乙醇中与氢氧化钠反应制备其钠盐。在磺胺结构中存在两个氨基,乙酰化时存在选择性问题,可生成双乙酰化产物,因此反应的pH值控制很重要,该合成路线的关键是选择性控制,以及反应终产物的分离和结晶。

反应产物及副产物在不同pH时的溶解情况见表5-1。反应产物及副产物在实验过程中随溶液酸碱性溶解和析出的过程如图5-2所示,操作时注意将滤液和滤饼分清楚。

表 5-1　磺胺醋酰及原料、副产物的溶解度

| 名称 | pH=7 | pH=4~5 | pH<2 |
| --- | --- | --- | --- |
| 磺胺 | 溶解度极小 | 溶 | 溶 |
| 磺胺醋酰 | 溶 | 溶解度低 | 溶 |
| 双乙酰化产物 | 溶 | 溶解度低 | 不溶 |

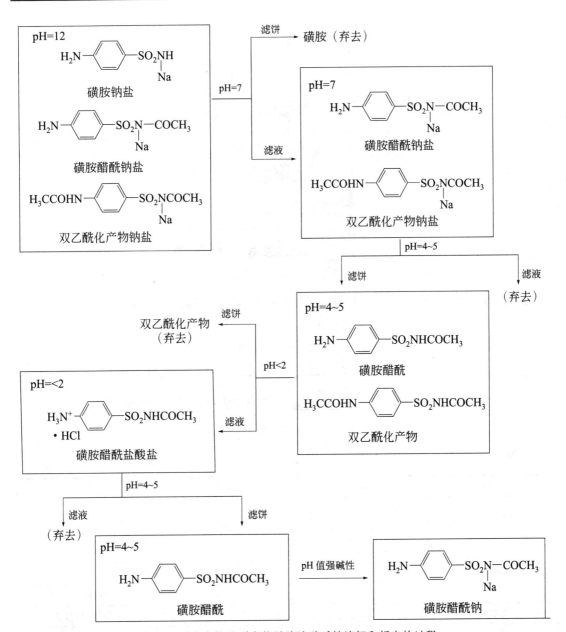

图 5-2　反应产物及副产物随溶液酸碱性溶解和析出的过程

安全提示：与其他腐蚀性酸和碱一样，氢氧化钠溶液接触皮肤后易导致化学灼伤，并且在与眼睛接触时可能引起永久失明。因此，在使用时，应始终使用防护设备，如佩戴橡胶手套、防护服和护目镜等。若不慎皮肤接触，应立即用水冲洗至少 15 min。

## Ⅲ 实验装置和原料

### 1. 实验装置

回流实验装置如图 5-3 所示。该装置由三颈烧瓶、球形冷凝管、磁力搅拌器和温度计等组成。

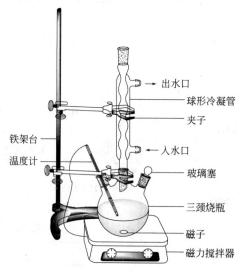

图 5-3　回流实验装置

碱化实验装置如图 5-4 所示。该装置主要由磁力搅拌器和烧杯等组成。

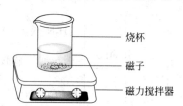

图 5-4　碱化实验装置

### 2. 原料

| 原材料名称 | 用量 | 规格 | 用途 |
|---|---|---|---|
| 磺胺 | 17.2 g（0.1 mol） | C. P. | 原料 |
| 醋酐 | 13.6 mL（0.14 mol） | C. P. | 乙酰化试剂 |
| 氢氧化钠溶液 | 22 mL（0.11 mol） | 22.5% | 原料 |
| | 12.5 mL（0.19 mol） | 77% | 原料 |
| | 适量 | 40% | 调反应体系 pH 值 |
| 浓盐酸 | 适量 | — | 调节体系 pH 值 |
| 稀盐酸 | 适量 | 10% | 溶解沉淀 |
| 活性炭 | 少量 | — | 脱色 |
| 氢氧化钠乙醇溶液 | 适量 | 5% | 成盐 |
| 水 | 适量 | — | 稀释 |

## Ⅳ 实验操作

### 1. 磺胺醋酰的制备

（1）按图 5-3 所示搭建回流实验装置。于 100 mL 三颈烧瓶中，投入原料磺胺 17.2 g、22.5% 氢氧化钠溶液 22 mL，开动搅拌，于水浴上加热至 50 ℃左右。

（2）待物料溶解后，滴加醋酐 3.6 mL，5 min 后滴加 77% 的氢氧化钠溶液 2.5 mL，保持反应液 pH 在 12~13 之间，随后每隔 5 min 交替滴加醋酐和氢氧化钠溶液，每次 2 mL，加料期间，反应温度维持在 50~55 ℃，pH 值维持 12~13。

（3）加料完毕，继续保温搅拌反应 30 min。

（4）将反应液转入 100 mL 烧杯，加水 20 mL 稀释。用浓盐酸调 pH 值至 7，于冰浴中放置 20~30 min，冷却析出固体。

（5）抽滤固体，用适量冰水洗涤。将洗液与滤液合并后用浓盐酸调 pH 值至 4~5，滤取沉淀压干。

（6）沉淀用 3 倍量的 10% 的盐酸溶解，放置 30 min，抽滤除去不溶物，滤液加少量活性炭室温脱色后，抽滤，滤液用 40% 的氢氧化钠溶液调 pH 值至 5，析出磺胺醋酰，抽滤，于红外灯下干燥，测熔点，称重。

（7）如熔点不合格，用热水（1∶15）精制。

### 2. 磺胺醋酰钠的制备

（1）按图 5-4 所示搭建碱化实验装置。将以上所得的磺胺醋酰投入 100 mL 烧杯中，加入 4 倍量 5% 氢氧化钠乙醇溶液，室温搅拌至固体完全溶解，即有大量固体析出，抽滤，得到磺胺醋酰钠。

（2）烘干纯品，称重，计算收率，测熔点。

（3）将产物送到指导教师指定的产品回收处。

## Ⅴ 实验结果

### 1. 磺胺醋酰钠收率

（1）计算磺胺醋酰钠的理论产量

$$磺胺————磺胺醋酰钠$$
$$M_w=172.21 \text{ g/mol}————M_w=254.24 \text{ g/mol}$$
$$0.1 \text{ mol}————0.1 \text{ mol}$$
$$理论产量=0.1 \text{ mol}×254.24 \text{ g/mol}=25.42 \text{ g}$$

（2）计算磺胺醋酰钠的收率

$$收率=\frac{产品实际产量}{产品理论产量}×100\%=\frac{(\quad)}{25.42 \text{ g}}×100\%=(\quad)\%$$

### 2. 产品外观与熔点

A. 外观：_____；

B. 熔点：

理论值：179~184 ℃

实测值：_____。

**3. 实验结果分析**

_____
_____
_____
_____
_____
_____
_____
_____。

# Ⅵ 注意事项

1. 本实验中使用氢氧化钠溶液有多种不同浓度，实验中切勿用错。

2. 滴加醋酐和氢氧化钠溶液是交替进行，每滴完一种溶液后，让其反应 5 min 后，再滴入另一种溶液。滴加使用玻璃吸管加入，滴加速度以一滴一滴滴下为宜。

3. 反应中保持反应液 pH 值在 12～13 很重要，否则收率会降低。

4. 不同 pH 条件下析出固体成分不同，切勿混淆。

# Ⅶ 思考题

1. 反应过程中，pH＝7 时析出的固体是什么？pH＝5 时析出的固体是什么？在 10％盐酸中的不溶物是什么？

2. 反应过程中，调节 pH＝12～13 是非常重要的，碱性过强或过弱会产生怎样的结果？

（丁丽娜）

# Experiment 6

# Synthesis of Benzocaine

## Background

Benzocaine is a topical anesthetic used for traumatic analgesia, ulcer pain, general itch, etc. It is not suitable for children at 2 years old or under 2 years old. It can only be used for the 2 years old under the advice and guidance of a professional doctor after fully weighing the advantages and disadvantages under special circumstances. Benzocaine can also be used as a cosmetic ultraviolent radiation absorber. The chemical structure of benzocaine is shown in Fig. 6-1.

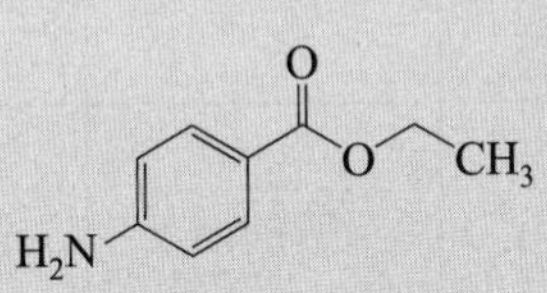

Fig. 6-1    Structure of Benzocaine

The local anesthetic (LA) drugs could prevent and relieve pain by interrupting nerve excitation and conduction by direct interaction with voltage-gated $Na^+$ channels to block the $Na^+$ current. As one of the most used LA drugs, benzocaine could also bind to the voltage-gated $Na^+$ channels, and thus block the channels to prevent and relieve pain. The full length X-ray crystal structures of human voltage-gated $Na^+$ channels have not been determined, but there are some crystal structures of voltage-gated $Na^+$ channels expressed in other animals like electric eel (PBD: 5XSY) or american cockroach. The homology modeled structure of human voltage-gated $Na^+$ channel was build and benzocaine was found to be well docked into the active pocket (**Color Diagram 6**). The binding site consists of a series hydrophobic residues, hence increasing hydrophobicity of LA drugs which in turn enhances the anesthetic effect. But the too large liposolubility is bad for LA drug to pass through the cell membrane.

# I  Purposes and Requirements

1. To master the synthesis of benzocaine by this experiment.

2. To master the principle and technology of oxidation reaction, esterification reaction and reduction reaction.

3. To understand the interaction between benzocaine and target.

# II  Principle of the Reaction

## 1. Physical data of the main reactants and product

| Name | Structure /CAS No. | Formula /M. Wt | b. p. or m. p. /℃ | Solubility |
|---|---|---|---|---|
| p-Nitrotoluene | 99-99-0 | $C_7H_7NO_2$ 137.13 | m. p. 51.7 | Do not dissolve in water; soluble in ethanol, ether, chloroform and benzene |
| p-Nitrobenzoic acid | 62-23-7 | $C_7H_5NO_4$ 167.13 | m. p. 237~240 | Slightly soluble in water; soluble in organic solvents such as ethanol |
| Ethyl p-nitrobenzoate | 99-77-4 | $C_9H_9NO_4$ 195.17 | m. p. 56~59 | Soluble in ethanol and ether; insoluble in water |
| Benzocaine | 94-09-7 | $C_9H_{11}NO_2$ 165.19 | m. p. 88~90 | Soluble in ethanol, ether and chloroform |
| Sodium dichromate dihydrate | $Na_2Cr_2O_7 \cdot 2H_2O$ 7789-12-0 | $Na_2Cr_2O_7 \cdot 2H_2O$ 297.85 | m. p. 357 (anhydrous) | Soluble in water, aqueous solution is acidic; insoluble in ethanol |
| Concentrated sulfuric acid | $H_2SO_4$ 7664-93-9 | $H_2SO_4$ 97.96 | — | More than mass fraction of 70% pure $H_2SO_4$ aqueous solution |
| Iron powder | Fe 7439-89-6 | Fe 55.84 | m. p. 1537 | — |

## 2. Synthetic route

$p$-Nitrotoluene     $p$-Nitrobenzoic acid

Ethyl $p$-nitrobenzoate     Benzocaine

The synthesis of benzocaine is started from $p$-nitrotoluene as a raw material. The first step is the oxidation of $p$-nitrotoluene by sodium dichromate to produce $p$-nitrobenzoic acid. The second step is esterification reaction catalyzed by sulfuric acid to prepare ethyl $p$-nitrobenzoate. The target product benzocaine is finally obtained by reducing $p$-nitrobenzoate with iron powder.

**Safety Tips:** Concentrated sulfuric acid, glacial acetic acid, sodium hydroxide and other strong acid and alkali reagents will be touched in this experiment. It should be noted that all the operation must be in ventilation. Strict compliance of operating procedures must be obeyed. You should also wear protective rubber gloves. When diluting or preparing an acid solution, acid was added to the water to avoid boiling and splashing. If sulfuric acid drops on your hand accidentally, you should immediately rinse your hand with plenty of water, and coat your hand with about 3% sodium bicarbonate solution. After the first aid treatment, you should go quickly to the nearby hospital for burn treatment to avoid further damage to the skin. If your skin contact with sodium hydroxide, you should rinse skin with water for at least 15 minutes (dilute solution) or wipe your skin with dry cloth (concentrate), then rinse skin with 5%~10% magnesium sulfate, or 3% boric acid solution and then go to hospital for further medical treatment. If your skin comes in contact with glacial acetic acid, you should first rinse your skin with water, and then thoroughly wash your skin with soap. If glacial acetic acid splashes into your eye, you should first rinse your eye with water, then wipe with a dry cloth. If the situation is serious, you need to go to hospital for medical treatment.

## Ⅲ  Experimental Equipments and Raw Materials

### 1. Experimental equipments

Oxidation reaction experimental set-up, Fig. 6-2, is composed from constant temperature magnetic stirrer, three-neck round-bottom flask, spherical condenser tube, thermometer and constant pressure dropping funnel.

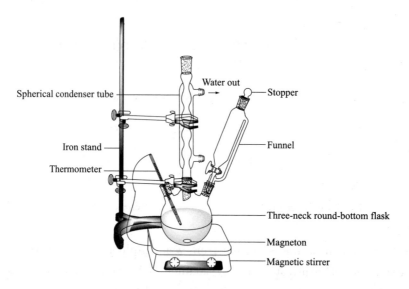

Fig. 6-2    Oxidation reaction experimental set-up

Esterification experimental set-up, Fig. 6-3, is composed from constant temperature magnetic stirrer, three-neck round-bottom flask, spherical condenser tube, thermometer and drying tube.

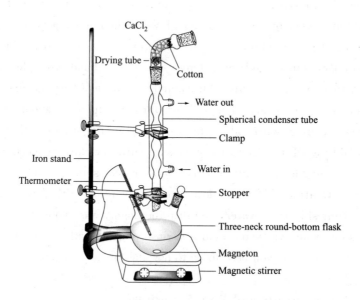

Fig. 6-3    Esterification experimental set-up

Reduction experimental set-up, Fig. 6-4, is composed from mechanical stirrer, three-neck round-bottom flask, spherical condenser tube, constant temperature magnetic stirrer and thermometer.

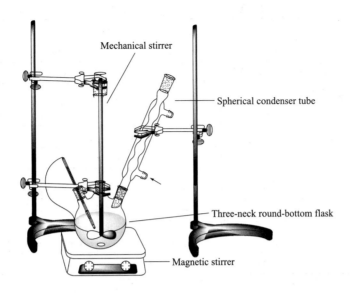

Mechanical stirrer

Spherical condenser tube

Three-neck round-bottom flask

Magnetic stirrer

Fig. 6-4　Reduction experimental set-up

## 2. Raw materials

| Synthetic product | Raw materials | | | |
|---|---|---|---|---|
| | Name | Quantity | Quality | Use |
| $p$-Nitrobenzoic acid | $Na_2Cr_2O_7 \cdot 2H_2O$ | 23. 6 g (0. 08 mol) | C. P. | Oxidant |
| | Distilled water | 130 mL | — | Solvent |
| | $p$-Nitrotoluene | 8 g (0. 06 mol) | C. P. | Reactant |
| | Concentrated sulfuric acid | 32 mL | C. P. | Catalyst |
| | 5% NaOH solution | 90 mL | — | Adjusting pH |
| | Activated carbon | 0. 5 g | — | Discolouring agent |
| | 5% Sulfuric acid | 70 mL | — | Reductant |
| Ethyl $p$-nitrobenzoate | $p$-Nitrobenzoic acid | 6 g (0. 036 mol) | Product prepared | Reactant |
| | Concentrated sulfuric acid | 2 mL | C. P. | Catalyst |
| | Distilled water | 100 mL | — | Solvent |
| | 5% $Na_2CO_3$ solution | 10 mL | — | Adjusting pH |
| | Absolute ethanol | 24 mL | A. R. | Solvent |
| Ethyl $p$-aminobenzoate（A） | Ethyl $p$-nitrobenzoate | 6 g (0. 031 mol) | Product prepared | Reactant |
| | Distilled water | 35 mL | — | Solvent |
| | Glacial acetic acid | 2. 5 mL | C. P. | Adjusting pH |
| | Iron powder | 8. 6 g (0. 154 mol) | particle size: 80 mesh | Reductant |
| | 95% Ethanol | 35 mL | — | Solvent |
| | $Na_2CO_3$ saturated solution | 3 g dissolved in 30 mL water | — | Adjusting pH |
| | 50% Ethanol | 10~15 mL/g | — | Solvent |

| Synthetic product | Raw materials | | | |
| --- | --- | --- | --- | --- |
| | Name | Quantity | Quality | Use |
| Ethyl p-aminobenzoate (B) | Ethyl p-nitrobenzoate | 5 g (0.026 mol) | Product prepared | Reactant |
| | Distilled water | 25 mL | — | Solvent |
| | NH₄Cl | 0.7 g | C. P. | Catalyst |
| | Iron powder | 4.3 g (0.077 mol) | particle size: 80 mesh | Reductant |
| | 5% Na₂CO₃ solution | Proper amount | — | Adjusting pH |
| | Chloroform | 40 mL | — | Solvent |
| | 5% hydrochloric acid | 90 mL | — | Adjusting pH |
| | 40% NaOH solution | Proper amount | — | Adjusting pH |
| Purification | Crude product | 3 g (0.018 mol) | Product prepared | Reactant |
| | 50% Ethanol | 10~15 mL/g | — | Solvent |

## IV  Operations

### 1. Preparation of p-nitrobenzoic acid

（1）Equip the oxidation reaction experimental set-up as shown in Fig. 6-2. Add 23.6 g sodium dichromate （$Na_2Cr_2O_7 \cdot 2H_2O$）and 50 mL water into the 250 mL three-necked round-bottom flask. Then, stir the solution until sodium dichromate is dissolved completely.

（2）Add 8 g p-nitrotoluene and then 32 mL concentrated sulfuric acid dropwise to the flask through the dropping funnel. After the concentrated sulfuric acid is added, start heating to maintain the reaction faint boiling for 60 minutes. There may be white crystal of nitrotoluene precipitation in the condenser. Hence, you should turn down the condensed water to make it melt and drip.

（3）After the solution is cooled, pour the mixture into a 250 mL breaker containing 80 mL of cold water. After vacuum filtration, wash the filter cake with water until the filtrate is colorless. Dissolve the resulting filter cake with 90 mL of 5% sodium hydroxide warm solution. Filter the mixture by suction at 50 °C. Add 0.5 g of activated carbon to the filtrate and stir the mixture for 5 ~ 10 minutes. Remove the activated carbon by hot vacuum filtration.

（4）After cooling, slowly pour the filtrate into 70 mL 5% sulfuric acid with full stirring. Following vacuum filtration, wash the solid with water. Dry the product under infrared lamp and weigh it up.

### 2. Preparation of ethyl p-nitrobenzoate (esterification)

（1）Equip the esterification experimental set-up as shown in Fig. 6-3. Add 6 g p-Nitrobenzoic acid and 24 mL of anhydride ethanol into dry 100 mL three-necked round-bottom flask. Next, slowly add 2 mL of concentrated sulfuric acid and shake the flask to mix evenly. Heat the solution to reflux for 80 minutes.

（2）When the solution is slightly cold, pour the reaction solution into a breaker containing

100 mL of water with stirring. Collect the solid by vacuum filtration.

(3) Transfer the residue to a mortar. Grind it finely and add 10 mL 5% sodium carbonate solution. Grind it for another 5 minutes, and check the pH value (pH should be > 7). After vacuum filtration, wash the solid mass with water. Dry the product under infrared lamp and weigh it up.

### 3. Preparation of ethyl p-aminobenzoate (reduction)

**Method A:**

(1) Equip the reduction experimental set-up as shown in Fig. 6-4. Add 35 mL water, 2.5 mL glacial acetic acid and 8.6 g iron powder into the 250 mL three-necked round-bottom flask.

(2) Stir the solution and heat at 95~98 ℃ for 5 minutes. When the solution is slightly cooled, add 6 g ethyl p-nitrobenzoate and 35 mL 95% ethanol. Reflux the solution for 90 minutes with vigorous stirring.

(3) When the solution is slightly cooled, gradually add warm saturated sodium carbonate solution (3 g sodium carbonate in 30 mL water). After the solution is stirred for a moment, remove the solid by vacuum filtration (Buchner funnel should be preheated). When the filtrate is cold, collect the precipitate by vacuum filtration. Wash the product with dilute ethanol. Dry the product under infrared lamp and weigh it up.

**Method B:**

(1) Equip the reduction experimental set-up as shown in Fig. 6-4. Add 25 mL water and 0.7 g ammonium chloride into the 250 mL three-necked round-bottom flask. Heat the solution to 95 ℃ and add 4.3 g iron powder quickly. Stir the solution for 5 minutes at 95~98 ℃.

(2) Quickly add 5 g ethyl p-aminobenzoate to the solution and stir it for 70 minutes at 95~98 ℃. Let the solution cool to 40 ℃.

(3) Adjust the pH of the solution to 7~8 by adding a small amount of saturated sodium carbonate solution. Add 30 mL chloroform to the solution and stir for 3~5 minutes. After vacuum filtration, wash three-necked round-bottom flask and residue by adding 10 mL chloroform. Pour the filtrate into a 100 mL separatory funnel. Discard the aqueous layer and extract the chloroform layer three times with 5% hydrochloric acid (30 mL×3). Adjust the pH of the pooled organic extracts 8 with 40% sodium hydroxide and precipitate the crystals. Crude benzocaine is obtained by vacuum filtration. Dry the product under infrared lamp and weigh it up.

### 4. Purification

(1) The crude product is recrystallized from 50% ethanol (10~15 mL/g) to give pure benzocaine. The product is dried under infrared lamp. Weigh the pure product and check the melting point.

(2) The reduction yield and total yield are calculated.

(3) Send the finished product to the place where the guide teachers designated.

## Ⅴ Experimental Results

### 1. Yield

(1) Calculate the theoretical production of benzocaine

$$p\text{-Nitrotoluene} \text{———} \text{Benzocaine}$$
$$M_w = 137.13 \text{ g/mol} \text{———} M_w = 165.19 \text{ g/mol}$$
$$0.06 \text{ mol} \text{———} 0.06 \text{ mol}$$
$$\text{Theoretical production} = 0.06 \text{ mol} \times 165.19 \text{ g/mol} = 9.91 \text{ g}$$

(2) Calculate the percent yield of benzocaine

$$\text{Yield} = \frac{\text{Practical production}}{\text{Theoretical production}} \times 100\% = \frac{(\quad)}{9.91 \text{ g}} \times 100\% = (\quad)\%$$

## 2. Appearance and melting point of product

A. Appearance: _____ ;

B. m. p. :

    Theoretical value: 88~90 ℃

    Practical value: _____ .

## 3. Analysis of experimental results

_____

_____

_____

_____

_____

_____

_____ .

## Ⅵ  Notes

1. In the oxidation reaction, when the residue was treated with 5% sodium hydroxide, the temperature should be maintained at about 50 ℃. When the temperature is low, sodium $p$-nitrobenzoate will precipitate and be filtered off.

2. Esterification reaction must be carried out under anhydrous conditions. If water goes into the reaction system, the yield will be reduced. Requirements of anhydrous operation include: 1) dry raw materials, 2) dry instrument and measuring cup, and 3) avoiding water goes into the reaction flask during the reaction.

3. Ethyl $p$-nitrobenzoate and a small amount of unreacted $p$-nitrobenzoic acid are dissolved in ethanol, but not soluble in water. When the reaction is completed, the solution is poured into water. When the concentration of ethanol is diluted, ethyl $p$-nitrobenzoate and $p$-nitrobenzoic acid will precipitate. This method of separation for this product is called dilution method.

4. Due to the high density of iron powder it is easy to sink in the bottom of the bottle, it must be stirred up in order to make the reaction smooth in the reduction reaction. One important factor in the reduction of iron powder is vigorous stirring. Iron powder in method A needs treatment. The method of iron treatment is as follows: add 10 g iron powder and 25 mL 2% hydrochloric acid to a beaker. Heat the solution to faint boiling. Obtain the solid

iron by suction filtration and wash until pH of the solution is $5 \sim 6$. The final iron powder product is obtained by drying.

5. The whole reaction takes place in a sequence whereby the product of the one step will be used in the next step. So, the amount of reagent used should be calculated proportionally.

## Ⅶ Discussion Questions

1. When the oxidation reaction is completed, on which chemical properties did the separation of *p*-nitrobenzoic acid from the mixture depends?

2. Why water-free operation is needed in the esterification reaction?

(By En Zhang)

# 实验六
# 苯佐卡因的合成

## 背景知识

苯佐卡因（Benzocaine）为局部麻醉药，用于手术后创伤止痛、溃疡痛、一般性痒等，不适用于 2 岁及 2 岁以下儿童患者，特殊情况下经充分权衡利弊后在专业医师建议和指导下才可使用。此外，苯佐卡因也可用作化妆品中的紫外线吸收剂。苯佐卡因的化学结构式为如图 6-1 所示。

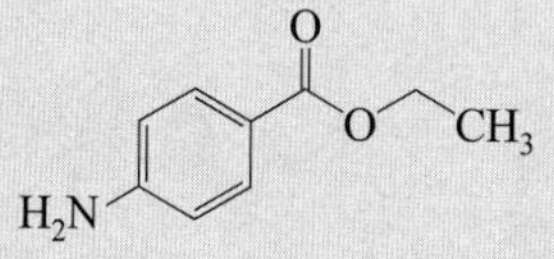

图 6-1 苯佐卡因的化学结构式

局部麻醉（local anesthetic，LA）药物通过与电压门控 $Na^+$ 通道直接相互作用阻断 $Na^+$ 电流，从而阻断神经兴奋和传导，进而预防和缓解疼痛。作为一种常用的局部麻醉药，苯佐卡因也能同电压门控 $Na^+$ 通道结合，阻断钠离子通道，从而预防和缓解疼痛。目前，尚无人源电压门控 $Na^+$ 通道的全长 X 射线衍射晶体结构被解析出来，但是已有一些动物的电压门控 $Na^+$ 通道的晶体结构，如电鳗（**彩插 6A**，PBD：5XSY）和美洲蟑螂。通过同源模建，我们得到了人源电压门控 $Na^+$ 通道的三维结构，计算研究发现通过分子对接苯佐卡因能较好地结合到电压门控 $Na^+$ 通道（**彩插 6B**）。由于结合位点是由一系列疏水氨基酸残基组成，因此增强化合物的疏水性可能提高麻醉效果，但当化合物脂溶性过大时，药物又难以穿越细胞膜。

## I  目的与要求

1. 通过本实验的操作，掌握苯佐卡因的合成。
2. 掌握氧化、酯化和还原的原理及实验操作。
3. 了解苯佐卡因与靶标的作用方式。

## Ⅱ 实验原理

### 1. 主要反应物及产物的物理常数

| 名称 | 结构式/CAS 号 | 分子式/分子量 | 沸点或熔点/℃ | 溶解度 |
|---|---|---|---|---|
| 对硝基甲苯 | （结构式）99-99-0 | $C_7H_7NO_2$ 137.13 | m. p. 51.7 | 不溶于水，易溶于乙醇、乙醚、氯仿和苯 |
| 对硝基苯甲酸 | （结构式）62-23-7 | $C_7H_5NO_4$ 167.13 | m. p. 237～240 | 微溶于水，能溶于乙醇等有机溶剂 |
| 对硝基苯甲酸乙酯 | （结构式）99-77-4 | $C_9H_9NO_4$ 195.17 | m. p. 56～59 | 易溶于乙醇和乙醚，不溶于水 |
| 苯佐卡因 | （结构式）94-09-7 | $C_9H_{11}NO_2$ 165.19 | m. p. 88～90 | 易溶于醇、醚、氯仿 |
| 重铬酸钠 | $Na_2Cr_2O_7 \cdot 2H_2O$ 7789-12-0 | $Na_2Cr_2O_7 \cdot 2H_2O$ 298.75 | m. p. 357 （无水） | 易溶于水，不溶于乙醇，水溶液呈酸性 |
| 浓硫酸 | $H_2SO_4$ 7664-93-9 | $H_2SO_4$ 97.96 | — | 指质量分数大于等于 70% 的纯 $H_2SO_4$ 的水溶液 |
| 铁粉 | Fe 7439-89-6 | Fe 55.84 | m. p. 1537 | — |

### 2. 合成路线

对硝基甲苯 $\xrightarrow[\text{浓}H_2SO_4]{Na_2Cr_2O_7}$ 对硝基苯甲酸 $\xrightarrow[\text{浓}H_2SO_4]{C_2H_5OH}$

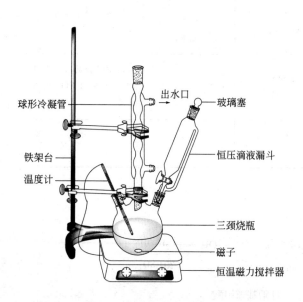

$$\text{对硝基苯甲酸乙酯} \xrightarrow{\text{Fe}} \text{苯佐卡因}$$

对硝基苯甲酸乙酯           苯佐卡因

以对硝基甲苯为原料，首先通过重铬酸氧化制备对硝基苯甲酸，然后在硫酸催化下在乙醇中反应制备对硝基苯甲酸乙酯，最后用铁粉还原得到苯佐卡因。

**安全提示**：本实验中会接触到浓硫酸、冰醋酸、氢氧化钠等强酸强碱试剂，在操作中注意通风，严格遵守操作规程，戴橡胶耐酸碱手套。稀释或制备酸溶液时，应把酸加入水中，避免沸腾和飞溅。如果不小心将硫酸滴在手上，立即用大量清水冲洗，并涂上浓度为3％左右的碳酸氢钠溶液，做完急救处理后，迅速到附近医院做灼伤处理，避免对皮肤进一步伤害。如果皮肤接触到氢氧化钠，先用水冲洗至少15 min（稀液）/用布擦干（浓液），再用5％～10％硫酸镁或3％硼酸溶液清洗并就医。若皮肤接触到冰醋酸先用水冲洗，再用肥皂彻底洗涤；若冰醋酸飞溅入眼睛，先用水冲洗，再用干布拭擦，情况严重的须送医院诊治。

## Ⅲ 实验装置和原料

### 1. 实验装置

氧化反应实验装置如图6-2所示。该装置主要包括三颈烧瓶、球形冷凝管、恒温磁力搅拌器、温度计和恒压滴液漏斗。

酯化反应实验装置如图6-3所示。该装置主要包括恒温磁力搅拌器、三颈烧瓶、球形冷凝管、温度计和干燥管。

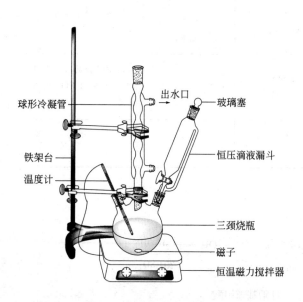

图6-2 氧化反应实验装置

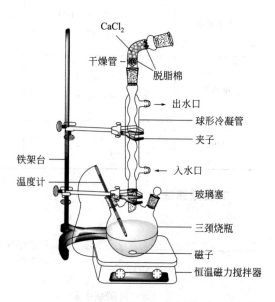

图6-3 酯化反应实验装置

铁粉还原实验装置如图 6-4 所示。该装置主要包括机械搅拌、三颈烧瓶、球形冷凝管、恒温磁力搅拌器、温度计。

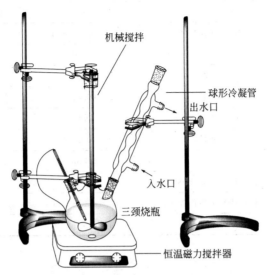

图 6-4　铁粉还原实验装置

## 2. 原料

| 合成产物 | 原料 | | | |
| --- | --- | --- | --- | --- |
| | 名称 | 用量 | 试剂级别 | 用途 |
| 对硝基苯甲酸 | 重铬酸钠（$Na_2Cr_2O_7 \cdot 2H_2O$） | 23.6 g（0.08 mol） | C. P. | 氧化剂 |
| | 蒸馏水 | 130 mL | — | 溶剂 |
| | 对硝基甲苯 | 8 g（0.06 mol） | C. P. | 原料 |
| | 浓硫酸 | 32 mL | C. P. | 催化剂 |
| | 5％氢氧化钠溶液 | 90 mL | | 调 pH 值 |
| | 活性炭 | 0.5 g | | 脱色 |
| | 5％硫酸 | 70 mL | | 调 pH 值 |
| 对硝基苯甲酸乙酯 | 对硝基苯甲酸 | 6 g（0.036 mol） | 自制 | 反应物 |
| | 浓硫酸 | 2 mL | C. P. | 催化剂 |
| | 蒸馏水 | 100 mL | — | 溶剂 |
| | 5％碳酸钠溶液 | 10 mL | | 调 pH 值 |
| | 无水乙醇 | 24 mL | 分析纯 | 溶剂 |
| 对氨基苯甲酸乙酯（A） | 对硝基苯甲酸乙酯 | 6 g（0.031 mol） | 自制 | 反应物 |
| | 蒸馏水 | 35 mL | — | 溶剂 |
| | 冰醋酸 | 2.5 mL | 化学纯 | 调 pH 值 |
| | 铁粉 | 8.6 g（0.154 mol） | 粒度：80 目 | 还原剂 |
| | 95％乙醇 | 35 mL | | 溶剂 |
| | 碳酸钠饱和溶液 | 3 g 溶于 30 mL 水 | | 调 pH 值 |
| | 50％乙醇 | 10～15 mL/g | — | 溶剂 |

| 合成产物 | 原料 | | | |
|---|---|---|---|---|
| | 名称 | 用量 | 试剂级别 | 用途 |
| 对氨基苯甲酸乙酯(B) | 对硝基苯甲酸乙酯 | 5 g (0.026 mol) | 自制 | 反应物 |
| | 蒸馏水 | 25 mL | — | 溶剂 |
| | 氯化铵 | 0.7 g | C. P. | 催化剂 |
| | 铁粉 | 4.3 g (0.077 mol) | 粒度:80目 | 还原剂 |
| | 5%碳酸钠溶液 | 适量 | — | 调 pH 值 |
| | 氯仿 | 40 mL | — | 溶剂 |
| | 5%盐酸 | 90 ml | — | 调 pH 值 |
| | 40%氢氧化钠 | 适量 | — | 调 pH 值 |
| 精制 | 对氨基苯甲酸乙酯粗品 | 3 g (0.018 mol) | 自制 | 原料 |
| | 50% 乙醇 | 10~15 mL/g | — | 溶剂 |

## Ⅳ 实验操作

**1. 对硝基苯甲酸的制备**

（1）按图 6-2 所示搭建氧化反应实验装置。于 250 mL 三颈烧瓶中，加入 23.6 g 重铬酸钠（含两个结晶水），50 mL 水，开动搅拌。

（2）待重铬酸钠溶解后加入 8 g 对硝基甲苯，搅拌均匀后用恒压滴液漏斗滴加 32 mL 浓硫酸，酸加完后开动加热，保持反应微沸 60 min（反应中，冷凝管中可能有白色针状的对硝基甲苯析出，可适当关小冷凝水，使它熔融滴下）。

（3）冷却后，将反应液倾入盛有 80 mL 冷水的 250 mL 烧杯中，抽滤，滤渣用水洗至滤液无色，所得滤渣溶于温热的 90 mL 5% 氢氧化钠溶液中，在 50 ℃ 左右抽滤，滤液加入 0.5 g 活性炭脱色（5~10 min），趁热抽滤。

（4）冷却后，在充分搅拌下，将滤液慢慢倒入 70 mL 5% 硫酸中，抽滤，洗涤，干燥得本品，计算收率。

**2. 对硝基苯甲酸乙酯的制备**

（1）按图 6-3 所示搭建酯化反应实验装置。在干燥的 100 mL 三颈烧瓶中加入 6 g 对硝基苯甲酸和 24 mL 无水乙醇，分三次加入 2 mL 浓硫酸，振摇使混合均匀，装上附有氯化钙干燥管的球形冷凝管，在油浴上加热回流 80 min。

（2）稍冷，在搅拌下，将反应液倾入 100 mL 水中，抽滤。

（3）滤渣移至乳钵中，研细后，加入 5% 碳酸钠溶液 10 mL，研磨 5 min，测 pH 值（检查反应物是否呈碱性），抽滤，用水洗涤，红外灯干燥得本品，计算收率。

**3. 对氨基苯甲酸乙酯的制备（还原）**

A 法：

（1）按图 6-4 所示搭建还原实验装置。在装有搅拌及球形冷凝管的 250 mL 三颈烧瓶中，加入 35 mL 水、2.5 mL 冰醋酸和已经处理过的 8.6 g 铁粉，开动搅拌。

（2）加热至 95 ~ 98 ℃，保持 5 min，稍冷，加入对硝基苯甲酸乙酯 6 g 和 95% 乙醇

35 mL，在剧烈搅拌下，回流 90 min。

（3）稍放冷，在搅拌下，分次加入温热的碳酸钠饱和溶液（由碳酸钠 3 g 和水 30 mL 配成），搅拌片刻后，立即抽滤（布氏漏斗需预热），在滤液冷却后析出结晶，抽滤，产品用稀乙醇洗涤，干燥得粗品。

B 法：

（1）按照图 6-4 所示搭建还原实验装置。在装有机械搅拌及球形冷凝管的 250 mL 三颈烧瓶中，加入 25 mL 水、0.7 g 氯化铵，加热至 95 ℃，快速加入 4.3 g 铁粉，95 ～ 98 ℃ 活化 5 min。

（2）快速加入 5 g 对硝基苯甲酸乙酯，在 95 ～ 98 ℃ 反应 70 min，冷却至 40 ℃ 左右。

（3）加入少量碳酸钠饱和溶液调至 pH = 7 ～ 8，加入氯仿 30 mL，搅拌 3～5 min，抽滤，用氯仿 7 ～ 10 mL 洗三颈烧瓶及滤渣，抽滤，将滤液倾入 100 mL 分液漏斗中，静置分层。水层放在一边，氯仿层用 5％盐酸 90 mL 分 3 次提取，合合提取液，用 40％氢氧化钠调至 pH = 8，析出结晶，抽滤，得苯佐卡因粗品。

**4. 精制**

（1）粗品用 50％ 乙醇（10 ～ 15 mL/ g）重结晶，得苯佐卡因。

（2）烘干纯品，称重，计算收率，测熔点。

（3）将产物送到指导教师指定的产品回收处。

# V 实验结果

**1. 收率**

（1）计算苯佐卡因的理论产量

$$对硝基甲苯 \text{————} 苯佐卡因$$

$$M_w = 137.13 \text{ g/mol} \text{————} M_w = 165.19 \text{ g/mol}$$

$$0.06 \text{ mol} \text{————} 0.06 \text{ mol}$$

$$理论产量 = 0.06 \text{ mol} \times 165.19 \text{ g/mol} = 9.91 \text{ g}$$

（2）计算苯佐卡因的收率

$$收率 = \frac{产品实际产量}{产品理论产量} \times 100\% = \frac{(\quad)}{9.91 \text{ g}} \times 100\% = (\quad)\%$$

**2. 产品外观与熔点**

A. 外观：＿＿＿＿＿＿＿＿＿＿＿＿＿＿＿＿＿＿＿＿＿；

B. 熔点：

　　理论值：88～90 ℃

　　实测值：＿＿＿＿＿＿＿＿＿＿＿＿＿＿＿＿＿。

**3. 实验结果分析**

＿＿＿＿＿＿＿＿＿＿＿＿＿＿＿＿＿＿＿＿＿＿＿＿＿＿＿＿＿＿＿＿＿＿＿＿＿＿＿＿

＿＿＿＿＿＿＿＿＿＿＿＿＿＿＿＿＿＿＿＿＿＿＿＿＿＿＿＿＿＿＿＿＿＿＿＿＿＿＿＿

＿＿＿＿＿＿＿＿＿＿＿＿＿＿＿＿＿＿＿＿＿＿＿＿＿＿＿＿＿＿＿＿＿＿＿＿＿＿＿＿

＿＿＿＿＿＿＿＿＿＿＿＿＿＿＿＿＿＿＿＿＿＿＿＿＿＿＿＿＿＿＿＿＿＿＿＿＿＿＿＿

_____

_____

_____·

## VI 注意事项

（1）在氧化反应中，用 5% 氢氧化钠处理滤渣时，温度应保持在 50 ℃左右，温度低，对硝基苯甲酸钠也会析出而被滤出。

（2）酯化反应必须在无水条件下进行，如有水进入反应系统中，收率将降低。无水操作的要求点是：1）原料干燥无水；2）所用仪器、量具干燥无水；3）反应期间避免水进入反应瓶中。

（3）对硝基苯甲酸乙酯及少量未反应的对硝基苯甲酸均溶于乙醇，但均不溶于水。反应完毕后，将反应物倾入水中，乙醇的浓度变稀，对硝基苯甲酸乙酯及对硝基苯甲酸便析出，这种分离产物的方法称为稀释法。

（4）在还原反应中，因铁粉密度大，沉于瓶底，必须将它搅拌起来，才能使反应顺利进行。充分剧烈搅拌是铁粉还原反应的重要因素。A 法中使用铁粉需要处理，其方法为：称取 10 g 铁粉，置于烧杯中，加入 2% 盐酸 25 mL，在石棉网上加热使之微沸，抽滤，水洗至 pH＝5 ～ 6，烘干，备用。

（5）整个反应是接着上一步反应进行的，所用试剂的量需要按照比例计算后使用。

## VII 思考题

1. 氧化反应完毕，依据哪些性质将对硝基苯甲酸从混合物中分离出来？
2. 酯化反应为什么需无水操作？

（张恩）

# Synthesis of Ciprofloxacin Monohydrochloride Monohydrate

## Background

Ciprofloxacin is a third generation quinolone antibiotics. It is developed and marketed by Bayer Pharmaceuticals in Germany and its commercial name is "Ciprobay". The chemical structure of ciprofloxacin is shown in Fig. 7-1.

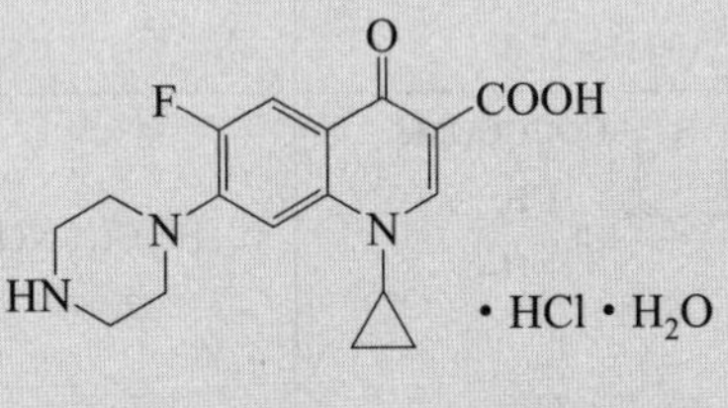

Fig. 7-1   Structure of ciprofloxacin

Subunit A of bacterial DNA gyrase is the target of ciprofloxacin and PDB: 2XCT was selected as the target protein. The crystal structure of ciprofloxacin and *Staphylococcus aureus* DNA gyrase are shown in **Color Diagram 7**. The binding pattern of ciprofloxacin is shown in **Color Diagram 7A.** Ciprofloxacin forms two hydrogen bonds with Ser 1084 and Arg 458, two coordination bonds with $Mn^{2+}$ and van der waals interaction with surrounding DNA bases. Therefore, it can stabilize the double strand breakage of DNA produced by DNA gyrase, inhibit the synthesis and replication of DNA, prevent cell division, and eventually lead to bacterial death and play a bactericidal role. The surface map of DNA gyrase of *Staphylococcus aureus*, ciprofloxacin and DNA complex crystal protein (**Color Diagram 7B**) clearly shows the binding site of ciprofloxacin on the A subunit of DNA gyrase.

# Ⅰ Purposes and Requirements

1. To master the principles and operation requirements of cyclization, hydrolysis and *N*-alkylation reaction.

2. To strengthen the anhydrous reaction operation.

3. To understand the interaction between ciprofloxacin hydrochloride and target.

# Ⅱ Principle of the Reaction

## 1. Physical data of the main reactants and product

| Name | Structure /CAS No. | Formula /M. Wt | b. p. or m. p. /℃ | Solubility |
|---|---|---|---|---|
| 2,4-Dichloro-5-fluoro-acetophenone | 704-10-9 | $C_8H_5Cl_2FO$ 207.03 | m. p. 33~36 | — |
| Methyl 3-(2,4-dichloro-5-fluorophenyl)-3-oxopropionate | 103319-17-1 | $C_{10}H_7Cl_2FO_3$ 265.07 | m. p. 158~161 | — |
| Methyl 3-(cyclopropylamino)-2-(2,4-dichloro-5-fluorobenzoyl)acrylate | 105392-26-5 | $C_{14}H_{12}Cl_2FNO_3$ 332.15 | m. p. 156~158 | — |
| 3-Quinolinecarboxylic acid, 7-chloro-1-cyclopropyl-6-fluoro-1,4-dihydro-4-oxo-,Methyl ester | 104599-90-8 | $C_{14}H_{11}ClFNO_3$ 295.69 | m. p. 256 | — |
| 7-Chloro-1-cyclopropyl-6-fluoro-1,4-dihydro-4-oxoquinoline-3-carboxylic acid | 86393-33-1 | $C_{13}H_9Cl_2FNO_3$ 281.67 | m. p. 245~246 | — |
| Ciprofloxacin | 85721-33-1 | $C_{17}H_{18}FN_3O_3$ 331.34 | m. p. 255~257 | — |

| Name | Structure /CAS No. | Formula /M. Wt | b. p. or m. p. /℃ | Solubility |
|---|---|---|---|---|
| Ciprofloxacin mono-hydrochloride monohydrate | (structure) 86393-32-0 | $C_{17}H_{18}FN_3O_3 \cdot$ $HCl \cdot H_2O$ 385.82 | m. p. 318~320 | Well soluble in water |
| Dimethyl carbonate | $(MeO)_2CO$ 616-38-6 | $C_3H_6O_3$ 90.08 | b. p. 90~91 | Miscible with eth-anol and ether; insol-uble in water |
| Sodium hydride | NaH 7646-69-7 | NaH 24.00 | m. p. 800 ℃ | Insoluble in or-ganic solvents; Easy to hydrolyze in moist air, and reacts vio-lently with water |
| Triethyl orthoformate | $HC(OEt)_3$ 122-51-0 | $C_7H_{16}O_3$ 148.20 | b. p. 146 | $H_2O$: 1.35 g/L |
| Acetic anhydride | (structure) 108-24-7 | $C_4H_6O_3$ 102.09 | b. p. 138~139 | Reaction with wa-ter to form acetic acid; Soluble in ether, chlor-oform and benzene |
| Cyclopropanamine | (structure) 765-30-0 | $C_3H_7N$ 57.09 | b. p. 49~50 | Miscible with wa-ter, ethanol and chlor-oform |
| Potassium carbonate | $K_2CO_3$ 584-08-7 | $K_2CO_3$ 138.21 | m. p. 891 | Well soluble in water |
| DMF | (structure) 68-12-2 | $C_3H_7NO$ 73.09 | b. p. 153 | Soluble in water and most organic solvents |
| Piperazine | (structure) 110-85-0 | $C_4H_{10}N_2$ 86.14 | m. p. 107~111 | Soluble in water, methanol and etha-nol; slightly soluble in benzene, ether |
| 3-Methyl-1-butanol | (structure) 123-51-3 | $C_5H_{12}O$ 88.15 | b. p. 132.5 | Slightly soluble in water; soluble in eth-anol, ether, benzene, chloroform and petro-leum ether; well solu-ble in acetone |

## 2. Synthetic route

F—(ring)—COMe, Cl, Cl  →(MeO)₂CO / NaH→  F—(ring)—COCH₂COOMe, Cl, Cl  →HC(OEt)₃ / ZnCl₂, Ac₂O→  [ F—(ring)—COCCOOMe ‖ CH OEt, Cl, Cl ]

**2,4-Dichloro-5-fluoroacetophenone**

**Methyl 3-(2,4-dichloro-5-fluorophenyl)-3-oxopropionate**

NH₂ (cyclopropyl) →

F—(ring)—COCCOOMe ‖ CH NH (cyclopropyl), Cl, Cl  →K₂CO₃ / DMF→  F—(quinoline ring)—COOMe, O, Cl, N-cyclopropyl  →(1) OH⁻ (2) H⁺→

**Methyl 3-(cyclopropylamino)-2-(2,4-dichloro-5-fluorobenzoyl)acrylate**

**3-Quinolinecarboxylic acid, 7-chloro-1-cyclopropyl-6-fluoro-1,4-dihydro-4-oxo-, Methyl ester**

F—(quinoline)—COOH, O, Cl, N-cyclopropyl  →(1) HN(piperazine)NH (2) isoamyl alcohol OH→  **Ciprofloxacin**

**7-Chloro-1-cyclopropyl-6-fluoro-1,4-dihydro-4-oxoquinoline-3-carboxylic acid**

→HCl, H₂O / CH₃CH₂OH→  **Ciprofloxacin monohydrochloride monohydrate** (· HCl · H₂O)

Methyl 3-(2,4-dichloro-5-fluorophenyl)-3-oxopropionate is obtained by $\beta$-keto-acid esterification from 2,4-dichloro-5-fluoroacetophenone, dimethyl carbonate and sodium hydride. Then, ciprofloxacin hydrochloride was synthesized by isomethylenization, cyclopropylamination, cyclization, hydrolysis, piperazine and salt formation.

**Safety Tips**: Gloves should be worn when acetic anhydride is used for it can cause severe burns. If it comes in contact with the skin, rinse it immediately with plenty of water.

Sodium hydride is stable in dry air and emits hydrogen when exposed to water which can cause fire.

Triethyl orthoformate is sensitive to water, flammable, volatile and irritating. It should be used in fume hood.

# Ⅲ Experimental Equipments and Raw Materials

## 1. Experimental equipments

Reaction experimental set-up （A）, Fig. 7-2, is composed from constant temperature magnetic stirrer, three-neck round-bottom flask, spherical condenser tube, thermometer, constant pressure dropping funnel and drying tube.

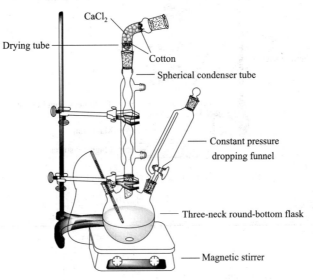

Fig. 7-2　Reaction experimental set-up （A）

Reaction experimental set-up （B）, Fig. 7-3, is composed from constant temperature magnetic stirrer, three-neck round-bottom flask, spherical condenser tube, thermometer and drying tube.

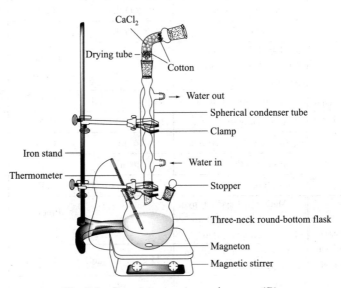

Fig. 7-3　Reaction experimental set-up （B）

Reaction experimental set-up (C), Fig. 7-4, is composed from constant temperature magnetic stirrer, three-neck round-bottom flask, spherical condenser tube and thermometer.

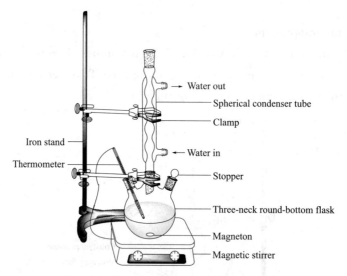

Fig. 7-4    Reaction experimental set-up (C)

## 2. Raw materials

| Synthetic product | Raw materials | | | |
| --- | --- | --- | --- | --- |
| | Name | Quantity | Quality | Use |
| Methyl 3-(2,4-dichloro-5-fluorophenyl)-3-oxopropionate | 2,4-Dichloro-5-fluoro-acetophenone | 10.8 g (0.05 mol) | ≥98% | Reactant |
| | NaH | 4.8 g (0.12 mol) | C. P. (60%) | Reactant |
| | Dimethyl carbonate | 13.5 g (0.15 mol) | C. P. | Reactant |
| | Toluene | 50 mL | C. P. | Solvent |
| | Glacial acetic acid | 20 mL | C. P. | Neutralization reagent |
| | Ice distilled water | 50 mL | C. P. | Hydrolysis agent |
| Methyl 3-(cyclopropylamino)-2-(2,4-dichloro-5-fluoro-benzoyl) acrylate | Methyl 3-(2,4-dichloro-5-fluorophenyl)-3-oxopropionate | 10 g | Product prepared | Reactant |
| | Triethyl orthoformate | 8.6 g (0.058 mol) | C. P. | Reactant |
| | Acetic anhydride | 10 g (0.097 mol) | C. P. | Reactant |
| | Zinc chloride anhydrous | 0.3 g | C. P. | Catalytic agent |
| | Absolute ethanol | 40 mL | C. P. | Solvent |
| | Cyclopropanamine | 2.5 g (0.044 mol) | C. P. | Reactant |
| 3-Quinolinecarboxylic acid, 7-chloro-1-cyclopropyl-6-fluoro-1,4-dihydro-4-oxo-,Methyl ester | Methyl 3-(cyclopropyl-amino)-2-(2,4-dichloro-5-fluorobenzoyl) acrylate | 5 g | Product prepared | Reactant |
| | Potassium carbonate anhydrous | 3.17 g (0.023 mol) | C. P. | Reactant |
| | DMF | 39 mL | C. P. | Solvent |
| | Water | 50 mL | — | Solid precipitation |

| Synthetic product | Raw materials | | | |
|---|---|---|---|---|
| | Name | Quantity | Quality | Use |
| 7-Chloro-1-cyclopropyl-6-fluoro-1,4-dihydro-4-oxoquinoline-3-carboxylic acid | 3-Quinolinecarboxylic acid, 7-chloro-1-cyclopropyl-6-fluoro-1,4-dihydro-4-oxo-, Methyl ester | Proper amount | Product prepared | Reactant |
| | Sodium hydroxide | 1.8 g (0.045 mol) | C. P. | Reactant |
| | Hydrochloric acid | Proper amount | C. P. | Adjusting pH |
| | Distilled water | 34 mL | — | Solvent |
| Ciprofloxacin monohydrochloride monohydrate | 7-Chloro-1-cyclopropyl-6-fluoro-1,4-dihydro-4-oxoquinoline-3-carboxylic acid | 4 g (0.014 mol) | Product prepared | Reactant |
| | Piperazine anhydrous | 4.8 g (0.056 mol) | C. P. | Reactant |
| | 3-Methyl-1-butanol | 30 mL | C. P. | Solvent |
| | 95% Ethanol | 50 mL | C. P. | Solvent |
| | Concentrated hydrochloric acid | Proper amount | C. P. | Reactant |
| | Distilled water | Proper amount | — | Solvent |
| | Activated carbon | 0.5 g | C. P. | Discolouring agent |

## Ⅳ  Operations

### 1. Preparation of methyl 3-(2,4-dichloro -5-fluorophenyl)-3-oxopropionate

(1) Equip the reaction experimental set-up (A) as shown in Fig. 7-2. Add 4.8 g sodium hydride, 13.5 g dimethyl carbonate and 50 mL toluene into the 250 mL three-neck round-bottom flask. Heat up the mixture to 40 ℃ and add 10.8 g 2,4-dichloro-5-fluoro-acetophenone dropwise. Control the rate to complete dropping within 15 minutes and keep the temperature below 75 ℃. Subsequently, raise the temperature to 75 ℃ and keep for 30 minutes, and then cool the the mixture to room temperature.

(2) Slowly add a mixture of glacial acetic acid (20 mL) and ice water (50 mL) to the above system dropwise. Dissolve the mixture by stirring and wait until layers are formed. Separate the organic layer and wash with water in three times.

(3) Recover the solvent to dry by rotary evaporation below 90 ℃, and a brown-red oil will be obtained. The oil will then solidify after cooling. Weigh the product and calculate the yield.

### 2. Preparation of methyl 3-(cyclopropylamino)-2-(2,4-dichloro -5-fluorobenzoyl) acrylate

(1) Equip the reaction experimental set-up (B) as shown in Fig. 7-3. Add 10 g ethyl 2,4-dichloro-5-fluorobenzoyl acetate, 8.6 g triethyl orthoformate, 10 g acetic anhydride and 0.3 g anhydrous zinc chloride into the 250 mL three-neck round-bottom flask and heat the mixture to reflux for 1 h.

(2) Recover the solvent to dry at a temperature below 110 ℃. A brown-red oil will be obtained.

(3) Add 40 mL anhydrous ethanol to the flask. Add cyclopropylamine (2. 5 g) dropwise for 20 minutes under the ice-water bath. And then, keep the reaction at room temperature for 1 h.

(4) Obtain the white crystals by filtration and drying. Dry the product under infrared lamp, weigh and measure the melting point.

### 3. Preparation of methyl 7-chloro-1-cyclopropyl-6-fluoro-4-oxo-1,4-dihydro-quinoline-3-carboxylate

(1) Equip the reaction experimental set-up (B) as shown in Fig. 7-3. Add 5 g methyl 3-(cyclopropylamino)-2-(2,4-dichloro-5-fluorobenzoyl) acrylate, 3. 17 g anhydrous potassium carbonate and 39 mL DMF into the 100 mL three-neck round-bottom flask. Heat up the mixture to 140 ℃ and keep for 1. 5 h.

(2) The mixture should be cooled to 50 ℃. Add 50 mL of water to the above reaction mixture, precipitate solid particles, filter and wash with water to obtain crude product. The crude product can be directly used in the next reaction.

### 4. Preparation of 7-chloro-1-cyclopropyl-6-fluoro-1,4-dihydro-4-oxoquinoline-3-carboxylic acid

(1) Equip the reaction experimental set-up (C) as shown in Fig. 7-4. A solution composed of above product, 1. 8 g sodium hydroxide and 34 mL distilled water are added to the 250 mL three-neck round-bottom flask and heated to 95~100 ℃ and maintain at this temperature for 1. 5 h. Then, cool the mixture is to 50 ℃. Adjust the pH to 1 with concentrated hydrochloric acid, raise the reaction temperature to 80 ℃ and maintain for 30 minutes, and cool to room temperature.

(2) Filter and wash the filtrate with water to neutralize the acid. Dry the product under infrared lamp. Weigh the product and calculate the yield. Measure the melting point. If the melting point does not match, recrystallization is needed.

(3) The recrystallization conditions are as follows: dissolve the crude product in 5 times DMF with heating. Add activated carbon and reheat. Filter while it is hot to remove activated carbon and crystallize by cooling. Filter it and wash the filtrate with DMF. Dry the product under infrared lamp.

### 5. Preparation of ciprofloxacin monohydrochloride monohydrate

(1) Equip the reaction experimental set-up (B) as shown in Fig. 7-3. Add 4 g of the product obtained above, 4. 8 g anhydrous piperazine and 30 mL 3-methyl-1-butanol into the 100 mL three-neck round-bottom flask. Heat up the mixture to reflux and maintain for 6 h. Cool the mixture to 10 ℃, precipitate the solid particles, filter and wash with water.

(2) Dissolve the solid product obtained in 20 mL of 10% hydrochloric acid, reflux with activated carbon for 30 minutes and filter while it is hot. Cool the filtrate to 65 ℃, add 95% ethanol, reflux to transparent, cool it again to 10~15 ℃, precipitate and filter.

(3) Dry the product under infrared lamp and weigh it up. Calculate the yield and measure the melting point.

(4) Send the final product to the place where the guide teachers designated.

## V Experimental Results

### 1. Yield

(1) Calculate the theoretical production of ciprofloxacin monohydrochloride mono-hydrate

2,4-Dichloro-5-fluoroacetophenone ——— Ciprofloxacin monohydrochloride monohydrate

$$M_w = 207.03 \text{ g/mol} \text{———} M_w = 385.82 \text{ g/mol}$$

$$0.05 \text{ mol} \text{———} 0.05 \text{ mol}$$

Theoretical production $= 0.05 \text{ mol} \times 385.82 \text{ g/mol} = 19.29 \text{ g}$

(2) Calculate the percent yield of ciprofloxacin monohydrochloride monohydrate

$$\text{Yield} = \frac{\text{Practical production}}{\text{Theoretical production}} \times 100\% = \frac{(\quad)}{19.29 \text{ g}} \times 100\% = (\quad)\%$$

### 2. Appearance and melting point of product

A. Appearance: _____ ;

B. m. p. :

Theoretical value: 318~320 ℃

Practical value: _____ .

### 3. Analysis of experimental results

_____

_____

_____

_____

_____

_____

_____ .

## VI Notes

1. The synthesis of methyl 3-(2,4-dichloro-5-fluorophenyl)-3-oxopropionate and methyl 3-(cyclopropylamino)-2-(2,4-dichloro-5-fluorobenzoyl) acrylate needs to be completed under completely anhydrous conditions. Otherwise, the yield will decrease.

2. The control of reaction temperature in each step is an important factor.

3. The whole reaction takes place in a sequence whereby the product of the one step will be used in the next step. So, the amount of reagent used should be calculated proportionally.

## VII Discussion Questions

1. Structurally, what substances can be used instead of sodium hydride?

2. Structurally，what substances can be used instead of Lewis acid $ZnCl_2$?

3. Structurally，what substances can be used instead of 3-methyl-butanol?

4. Structurally，what substances are the by-product of piperazine reaction of 6-fluoro in the condensation reaction of piperazine?

（By Wen Li，Hongmin Liu）

## 实验七
# 盐酸环丙沙星的合成

## 背景知识

环丙沙星（Ciprofloxacin），也称作环丙氟哌酸，为第三代喹诺酮类抗菌药物，由德国拜耳医药开发上市，商品名为"西普乐"，其化学结构式见图 7-1。

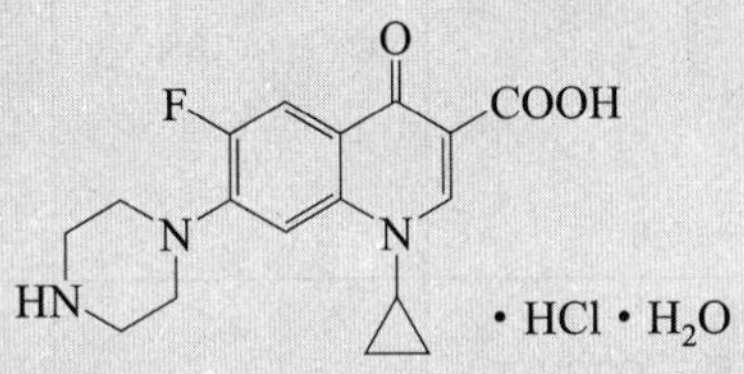

图 7-1　环丙沙星化学结构式

环丙沙星的作用靶标为细菌 DNA 回旋酶的 A 亚单位，选择 PDB：2XCT 为靶标蛋白进行分子模拟。**彩插 7** 是计算模拟环丙沙星和金黄色葡萄球菌 DNA 回旋酶作用模式图。环丙沙星的结合模式如**彩插 7A** 所示，环丙沙星与 Ser 1084、Arg 458 形成两个氢键，与 $Mn^{2+}$ 形成两个配位键，还与周围 DNA 碱基形成范德华相互作用。因此，可以稳定由 DNA 回旋酶产生的 DNA 双链断裂，从而抑制 DNA 的合成和复制，阻止细胞分裂，最终导致细菌死亡起到杀菌作用。金黄色葡萄球菌 DNA 回旋酶、环丙沙星和 DNA 复合晶体蛋白表面图（**彩插 7B**），清楚地显示了环丙沙星在 DNA 回旋酶的 A 亚基上的结合位点。

## Ⅰ　目的与要求

1. 掌握环合反应、水解反应、N-烷基化反应的原理和操作要求。
2. 进一步巩固无水反应操作。
3. 了解盐酸环丙沙星与靶标的作用方式。

## Ⅱ　实验原理

**1. 主要反应物和产物的物理常数**

| 名称 | 结构式/CAS 号 | 分子式/分子量 | 沸点或熔点/℃ | 溶解度 |
|---|---|---|---|---|
| 2,4-二氯-5-氟苯乙酮 | F COMe / Cl Cl / 704-10-9 | $C_8H_5Cl_2FO$ 207.03 | m. p. 33～36 | — |
| 2,4-二氯-5-氟苯甲酰乙酸甲酯 | F COCH$_2$COOMe / Cl Cl / 103319-17-1 | $C_{10}H_7Cl_2FO_3$ 265.07 | m. p. 158～161 | — |
| 2-(2,4-二氯-5-氟苯甲酰)-3-环丙氨基丙烯酸甲酯 | F COCCOOMe / CH / Cl Cl / NH / 105392-26-5 | $C_{14}H_{12}Cl_2FNO_3$ 332.15 | m. p. 156～158 | — |
| 1-环丙基-7-氯-6-氟-1,4-二氢-4-氧代喹啉-3-羧酸甲酯 | F O COOMe / Cl N / 104599-90-8 | $C_{14}H_{11}ClFNO_3$ 295.69 | m. p. 256 | — |
| 1-环丙基-7-氯-6-氟-1,4-二氢-4-氧代喹啉-3-羧酸 | F O COOH / Cl N / 86393-33-1 | $C_{13}H_9Cl_2FNO_3$ 281.67 | m. p. 245～246 | — |
| 环丙沙星 | F O COOH / HN N / 85721-33-1 | $C_{17}H_{18}FN_3O_3$ 331.34 | m. p. 255～257 | — |
| 盐酸环丙沙星 | F O COOH / HN N · HCl · H$_2$O / 86393-32-0 | $C_{17}H_{18}FN_3O_3$ · $HCl$ · $H_2O$ 385.82 | m. p. 318～320 | 易溶于水 |
| 碳酸二甲酯 | $(MeO)_2CO$ 616-38-6 | $C_3H_6O_3$ 90.08 | b. p. 90～91 | 能与乙醇和乙醚混溶,不溶于水 |
| 氢化钠 | NaH 7646-69-7 | NaH 24.00 | m. p. 800℃ | 不溶于有机溶剂;在潮湿空气中极易水解;遇水剧烈反应 |
| 原甲酸三乙酯 | $HC(OEt)_3$ 122-51-0 | $C_7H_{16}O_3$ 148.20 | b. p. 146 | 水:1.35 g/L |

| 名称 | 结构式/CAS号 | 分子式/分子量 | 沸点或熔点/℃ | 溶解度 |
|---|---|---|---|---|
| 乙酸酐 | $H_3C$—CO—O—CO—$CH_3$<br>108-24-7 | $C_4H_6O_3$<br>102.09 | b. p.<br>138～139 | 遇水反应,生成醋酸;易溶于乙醚、氯仿和苯 |
| 环丙胺 | $NH_2$—环丙基<br>765-30-0 | $C_3H_7N$<br>57.09 | b. p.<br>49～50 | 易溶于水、乙醇和氯仿 |
| 碳酸钾 | $K_2CO_3$<br>584-08-7 | $K_2CO_3$<br>138.21 | m. p.<br>891 | 易溶于水 |
| DMF | $H$—CO—$N(CH_3)_2$<br>68-12-2 | $C_3H_7NO$<br>73.09 | b. p.<br>153 | 和水及大部分有机溶剂互溶 |
| 无水哌嗪 | HN—哌嗪—NH<br>110-85-0 | $C_4H_{10}N_2$<br>86.14 | m. p.<br>107～111 | 溶于水、甲醇、乙醇,微溶于苯、乙醚 |
| 异戊醇 | (异戊醇结构)—OH<br>123-51-3 | $C_5H_{12}O$<br>88.15 | b. p.<br>132.5 | 微溶于水,可混溶于乙醇、乙醚、苯、氯仿、石油醚,易溶于丙酮 |

## 2. 合成路线

2,4-二氯-5-氟苯乙酮 —[$(MeO)_2CO$, NaH]→ 2,4-二氯-5-氟苯甲酰乙酸甲酯 —[$HC(OEt)_3$, $ZnCl_2$, $Ac_2O$]→ [中间体]

—[$NH_2$-环丙胺]→ 2-(2,4-二氯-5-氟苯甲酰)-3-环丙胺基丙烯酸甲酯 —[$K_2CO_3$, DMF]→ 1-环丙基-7-氯-6-氟-1,4-二氢-4-氧代喹啉-3-羧酸甲酯 —[(1) $OH^-$ (2) $H^+$]→

1-环丙基-7-氯-6-氟-1,4-二氢-4-氧代喹啉-3-羧酸 —[(1) HN—哌嗪—NH (2) 异戊醇]→ 环丙沙星

$$\xrightarrow[\text{CH}_3\text{CH}_2\text{OH}]{\text{HCl, H}_2\text{O}}$$

盐酸环丙沙星一水合物

2,4-二氯-5-氟苯乙酮、碳酸二甲酯与氢化钠发生 $\beta$-酮酸酯化生成 2,4-二氯-5-氟苯甲酰乙酸乙酯，然后，通过异氧亚甲基化、环丙胺化、关环、水解和哌嗪化和成盐反应得到盐酸环丙沙星。

**安全提示**：醋酸酐会引起严重烧伤，使用时应戴上手套，如果接触皮肤，立即用大量水冲洗。

氢化钠在干燥空气中稳定，遇水放出氢气，可引起着火。

原甲酸三乙酯对水气很敏感，易燃，具有较强的挥发性和刺激性气味，应该在通风橱中使用。

## Ⅲ 实验装置和原料

### 1. 实验装置

反应实验装置（A）见图 7-2 所示。该装置主要由磁力搅拌器、三颈烧瓶、球形冷凝管、温度计、恒压滴液漏斗和干燥管组成。

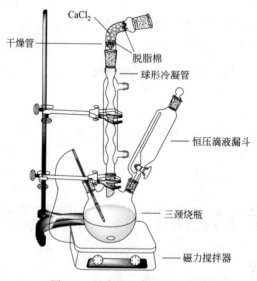

图 7-2 反应实验装置（A）

反应实验装置（B）如图 7-3 所示，主要由磁力搅拌器、三颈烧瓶、球形冷凝管、温度计和干燥管组成。

反应实验装置（C）如图 7-4 所示，主要由磁力搅拌器、三颈烧瓶、球形冷凝管和温度计组成。

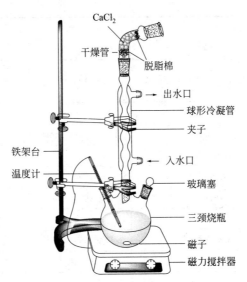

图 7-3　反应实验装置（B）

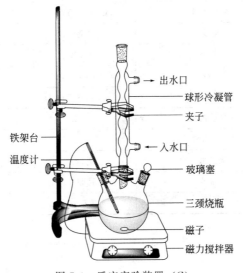

图 7-4　反应实验装置（C）

## 2. 原料

| 合成产物 | 原料 | | | |
| --- | --- | --- | --- | --- |
| | 名称 | 用量 | 试剂级别 | 用途 |
| 2,4-二氯-5-氟苯甲酰乙酸甲酯 | 2,4-二氯-5-氟苯乙酮 | 10.8 g(0.05 mol) | ≥98 % | 反应物 |
| | NaH | 4.8 g(0.12 mol) | 化学纯(60%) | 反应物 |
| | 碳酸二甲酯 | 13.5 g(0.15 mol) | 化学纯 | 反应物 |
| | 甲苯 | 50 mL | 化学纯 | 溶剂 |
| | 冰醋酸 | 20 mL | 化学纯 | 中和反应 |
| | 冰纯水 | 50 mL | 化学纯 | 水解剂 |

| 合成产物 | 原料 | | | |
|---|---|---|---|---|
| | 名称 | 用量 | 试剂级别 | 用途 |
| 2-(2,4-二氯-5-氟苯甲酰)-3-环丙胺基丙烯酸甲酯 | 2,4-二氯-5-氟苯甲酰乙酸乙酯 | 10 g | 自制 | 反应物 |
| | 原甲酸三乙酯 | 8.6 g (0.058 mol) | 化学纯 | 反应物 |
| | 乙酸酐 | 10 g (0.097 mol) | 化学纯 | 反应物 |
| | 无水氯化锌 | 0.3 g | 化学纯 | 催化剂 |
| | 无水乙醇 | 40 mL | 化学纯 | 溶剂 |
| | 环丙胺 | 2.5 g (0.044 mol) | 化学纯 | 反应物 |
| 1-环丙基-7-氯-6-氟-1,4-二氢-4-氧代喹啉-3-羧酸甲酯 | 环丙胺化物 | 5 g | 自制 | 反应物 |
| | 无水碳酸钾 | 3.17 g (0.023 mol) | 化学纯 | 反应物 |
| | DMF | 39 mL | 化学纯 | 溶剂 |
| | 水 | 50 mL | — | 析出固体 |
| 1-环丙基-7-氯-6-氟-1,4-二氢-4-氧代喹啉-3-羧酸 | 环化物 | 适量 | 自制 | 反应物 |
| | 氢氧化钠 | 1.8 g (0.045 mol) | 化学纯 | 反应物 |
| | 盐酸 | 适量 | 化学纯 | 调节 pH 值 |
| | 蒸馏水 | 34 mL | — | 溶剂 |
| 盐酸环丙沙星 | 环丙羧酸 | 4 g (0.014 mol) | 自制 | 反应物 |
| | 无水哌嗪 | 4.8 g (0.056 mol) | 化学纯 | 反应物 |
| | 异戊醇 | 30 mL | 化学纯 | 溶剂 |
| | 95 % 乙醇 | 50 mL | 化学纯 | 溶剂 |
| | 浓盐酸 | 适量 | 化学纯 | 反应物 |
| | 蒸馏水 | 适量 | — | 溶剂 |
| | 活性炭 | 0.5 g | 化学纯 | 脱色剂 |

## Ⅳ 实验操作

### 1. 2,4-二氯-5-氟苯甲酰乙酸甲酯合成

（1）按图 7-2 所示搭建反应实验装置（A）。在 250 mL 三颈烧瓶中，加入 4.8 g 氢化钠、13.5 g 碳酸二甲酯和 50 mL 甲苯，升温至 40 ℃，滴加 2,4-二氯-5-氟苯乙酮，控制滴加速度，15 min 滴完，滴加过程温度保持在 70 ℃以下。随后，75 ℃反应 30 min，冷却至室温。

（2）在以上体系中，缓慢滴加冰醋酸（20 mL）和冰水（50 mL）的混合物，搅拌至溶解，静置分层。分离有机层，水洗三次。

（3）90 ℃以下减压回收溶剂至干，得到棕红色油状物，冷却后固化，称重，计算收率。

### 2. 2-(2,4-二氯-5-氟苯甲酰)-3-环丙胺基丙烯酸甲酯合成

（1）按图 7-3 所示搭建反应实验装置（B）。在 250 mL 三颈烧瓶中，加入 10 g 2,4-二氯-5-氟苯甲酰乙酸乙酯、8.6 g 原甲酸三乙酯、10 g 乙酸酐和 0.3 g 无水氯化锌，升温至回流反应 1 h。

（2）110 ℃以下减压回收溶剂至干，得到棕红色油状物。

（3）向反应瓶中加入 40 mL 无水乙醇，冰水浴条件下，20 min 内滴加 2.5 g 环丙胺，室温反应 1 h。

（4）抽滤，干燥得白色晶体，测熔点，称重，计算收率。

**3.1-环丙基-7-氯-6-氟-1，4-二氢-4-氧代喹啉-3-羧酸甲酯合成**

（1）按图 7-3 所示搭建反应实验装置（B）。于 100 mL 三颈烧瓶中，加入 5 g 环丙胺化物、3.17 g 无水碳酸钾和 39 mL DMF，升温至 140 ℃反应 1.5 h。

（2）降温至 50 ℃，在以上体系中，加入 50 mL 水，析出固体，抽滤，水洗，得粗品。将粗品直接用于下一步反应。

**4.1-环丙基-7-氯-6-氟-1，4-二氢-4-氧代喹啉-3-羧酸合成**

（1）按图 7-4 所示搭建反应实验装置（C）。在 250 mL 三颈烧瓶中，加入环合物、1.8 g 氢氧化钠和 34 mL 蒸馏水配成的溶液，升温至 95～100 ℃反应 1.5 h，冷却至 50 ℃。然后，用浓盐酸调 pH＝1，升温至 80 ℃反应 0.5 h，冷却至室温。

（2）过滤，水洗至中性，烘干，测熔点（234～237 ℃）。若熔点不符，则需重结晶，计算收率。

（3）重结晶的条件为：取粗品，用 5 倍量的 DMF，加热溶解，加入活性炭，再次加热，过滤，除去活性炭，冷却，结晶，抽滤，洗涤，烘干得产品。

**5. 盐酸环丙沙星合成**

（1）按图 7-3 所示搭建反应实验装置（B）。100 mL 三颈烧瓶中，加入 4 g 环丙羧酸、4.8 g 无水哌嗪和 30 mL 异戊醇，升温至回流反应 6 h。冷却至 10 ℃，析出固体，抽滤，水洗。

（2）将所获得的固体溶于 10 ％盐酸 20 mL 中，加活性炭回流 0.5 h。热过滤，滤液冷却至 65 ℃，加入 95 ％乙醇，继续回流至透明，冷却至 10～15 ℃，析出固体，抽滤。

（3）烘干纯品，称重，计算收率，测熔点。

（4）将产物送到指导教师指定的产品回收处。


# V 实验结果


**1. 收率**

（1）计算盐酸环丙沙星的理论产量

$$2,4-二氯-5-氟苯乙酮 ——— 盐酸环丙沙星$$

$$M_w＝207.03 \text{ g/mol} ——— M_w＝385.82 \text{ g/mol}$$

$$0.05 \text{ mol} ——— 0.05 \text{ mol}$$

$$理论产量＝0.05 \text{ mol}×385.82 \text{ g/mol}＝19.29 \text{ g}$$

（2）计算盐酸环丙沙星的收率

$$收率＝\frac{产品实际产量}{产品理论产量}×100 ％＝\frac{(\qquad)}{19.29 \text{ g}}×100 ％＝(\qquad)％$$

**2. 产品外观与熔点**

A. 外观：＿＿＿＿＿＿＿＿＿＿＿；

B. 熔点：

    理论值：318～320℃

    实测值：＿＿＿＿＿＿＿＿＿＿＿。

**3. 实验结果分析**

_____

_____

_____

_____

_____

_____

_____ .

Ⅵ 注意事项

1. 2,4-二氯-5-氟苯甲酰乙酸乙酯和 2-(2,4-二氯-5-氟苯甲酰)-3-环丙胺基丙烯酸甲酯合成的反应需要在完全无水条件下完成，否则，反应收率下降。

2. 各步骤反应温度控制是重要的因素。

3. 整个反应是接着上一步反应进行的，所用试剂的量需要按照比例计算后使用。

Ⅶ 思考题

1. 用结构式表示，氢化钠还可以用什么代替？

2. 用结构式表示，所用 Lewis 酸 $ZnCl_2$ 还可以用什么代替？

3. 用结构式表示，所用异戊醇还可以用什么代替？

4. 哌嗪化反应时，6-氟发生哌嗪化的副产物的结构式是什么？

（李雯 刘宏民）

# Experiment 8

# Synthesis of Phenytoin Sodium

## Background

Phenytoin sodium, also known as dilantin, is a preferred antiepileptic drug for tonic-clonic seizures, and also be used as antiarrhythmic drug. The chemical structure of phenytoin sodium is shown in Fig. 8-1.

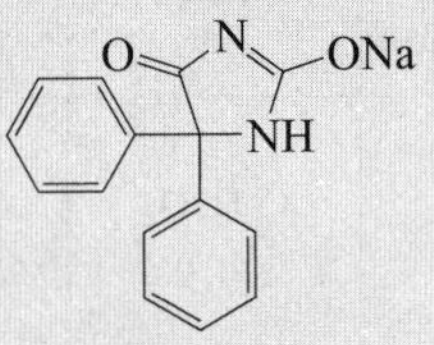

Fig. 8-1　Structure of Phenytoin Sodium

Voltage-gated sodium channels (VGSC) are the target for phenytoin and the PDB ID: 6AGF was choosen as the target protein. Predicted binding mode of phenytoin with VGSC was shown in **Color Diagram 8**. The binding pattern of phenytoin is shown in **Color Diagram 8A**, the amino group at position-4 of hydantoin forms a cation-$\pi$ interaction with the benzene group of residue Tyr 1593 residue, and the two benzene groups of phenytoin could form strong hydrophobic interactions with surrounding hydrophobic residues Phe 1601, Leu 443, Phe 805 and Tyr 1593. In addition, the one benzene group of phenytoin could form a $\pi$-$\pi$ stacking with the Phe 1601 residue, and the two benzene groups are almost at right angles to amide group and could also interact with other S6 segments to fill the inner pore of VGSC to prevent $Na^+$ permeation, thereby stabilizing the nerve cell membrane, and preventing the abnormal electrical activity of brain lesions from spreading to surrounding normal brain tissue, thus playing an anti-epileptic role. **Color Diagram 8B** clearly showed that phenytoin can stably bind to the active site of VGSC.

# Ⅰ Purposes and Requirements

1. To master the principle and operation requirements of benzoin condensation reaction, oxidation reaction and rearrangement reaction.

2. To understand the interaction between phenytoin sodium and target.

# Ⅱ Principle of the Reaction

## 1. Physical data of the main reactants and product

| Name | Structure/CAS No. | Formula /M. Wt | b. p. or m. p. /℃ | Solubility |
|---|---|---|---|---|
| Benzaldehyde | CHO  100-52-7 | $C_7H_6O$  106. 12 | b. p. 179 | Water: $<0.01$ g/100 mL |
| Benzoin | OH  O  119-53-9 | $C_{14}H_{12}O_2$  212. 24 | m. p. 134~138 | Insoluble in water, slightly soluble in ethers, soluble in ethanols |
| 1-Phenyl-1, 2-propanedione | O  O  579-07-7 | $C_9H_8O_2$  210. 23 | m. p. 95~96 | Soluble in ethanol, ether, acetone, benzene and chloroform; insoluble in water |
| Phenytoin | H  O  N  O  NH  57-41-0 | $C_{15}H_{12}N_2O_2$  252. 27 | m. p. 293~295 | In water: $<0.01$ g/100 mL; soluble in DMSO |
| Phenytoin sodium | O  N  ONa  NH  630-93-3 | $C_{15}H_{11}NaO_2$  274. 25 | m. p. 292~299 | Well soluble in water; soluble in ethanol; insoluble in chloroform |
| Thiamine hydro- chloride (Vitamin $B_1$) | $NH_2 \cdot HCl$  $Cl^-$  $N^+$  $H_3C$  $H_3C$  OH  67-03-8 | $C_{12}H_{16}N_4OS \cdot$ HCl 337. 27 | m. p. 245~250 | Well soluble in water; slightly soluble in ethanol; insoluble in ether, benzene, chloroform and acetone |
| Ferric chloride hexahydrate | $FeCl_3 \cdot 6H_2O$  10025-77-1 | $FeCl_3 \cdot 6H_2O$  270. 30 | m. p. 37 | Well soluble in water |
| Urea | $NH_2CONH_2$  57-13-6 | $CH_4N_2O$  60. 06 | m. p. 132. 7 | Soluble in water, methanol, formaldehyde, ethanol, solution ammonia and ethanol; slightly soluble in ether, chloroform, benzene |

## 2. Synthetic route

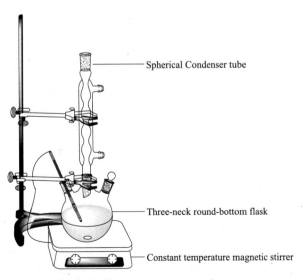

Benzaldehyde             Benzoin             1-Phenyl-1,2-propanedione

5,5-Diphenylhydantoin             Phenytoin sodium

Benzoin is obtained from benzaldehyde by benzoin condensation reaction which uses vitamin $B_1$ as a cofactor. Benzoin then undergoes oxidation to form 1,2-diphenylethylene ketone. Phenytoin is then synthesized by condensation and rearrangement reactions from urea in alkaline condition. Finally, sodium phenytoin is prepared by salt formation reaction.

**Safety Tips:** Benzaldehyde can stimulate the mucosa of the eyes and respiratory tract.

## Ⅲ Experimental Equipment and Raw Materials

### 1. Experimental equipment

Reaction experimental set-up, Fig. 8-2, is composed from constant temperature magnetic stirrer, three-neck round-bottom flask, spherical condenser tube and thermometer.

Fig. 8-2    Reaction experimental set-up

## 2. Raw materials

| Synthetic product | Raw materials | | | |
|---|---|---|---|---|
| | Name | Quantity | Quality | Use |
| Benzoin | Benzaldehyde | 10 mL (0.098 mol) | C. P. | Reactant |
| | Thiamine hydrochloride (Vitamin $B_1$) | 1.75 g(0.005 mol) | C. P. (60 %) | Catalytic agent |
| | 95 % ethanol | 15 mL | — | Solvent |
| | 2 mol/L NaOH | 5 mL | — | Catalytic agent |
| | Distilled water | Proper amount | — | Solvent |
| 1-Phenyl-1,2-propanedione | Benzoin | 2.12 g (0.010 mol) | Product prepared | Reactant |
| | Ferric chloride hexahydrate | 9.0 g (0.033 mol) | C. P. | Oxidizing agent |
| | Glacial acetic acid | 10 mL | C. P. | Solvent |
| | 95 % Ethanol | Proper amount | C. P. | Solvent |
| | Distilled water | Proper amount | — | Solvent |
| | Ethyl ether | Proper amount | C. P. | Solvent |
| Phenytoin | 1-Phenyl-1,2-propanedione | 1 g | Product prepared | Reactant |
| | Urea | 0.57 g (0.0095 mol) | C. P. | Reactant |
| | 15 % NaOH | 3.1 L | Product prepared | Catalytic agent |
| | 95 % Ethanol | 5 mL | C. P. | Solvent |
| | 15 % Hydrochloric acid | proper amount | — | Neutralization reagent |
| | Distilled water | 37 mL | | Solvent |
| Phenytoin sodium | Phenytoin | 1 g | Product prepared | Reactant |
| | 15 % NaOH | 5 mL | Product prepared | Reactant |
| | Activated carbon | Proper amount | C. P. | Discolouring agent |
| | Distilled water | 5 mL | — | Solvent |

## Ⅳ  Operations

### 1. Preparation of benzoin

（1）Equip the reaction experimental set-up as shown in Fig. 8-2. Add 1.75 g Vitamin $B_1$ and 4 mL distilled water into the 50 mL three-neck round-bottom flask，dissolve by stirring. Add 15 mL 95 % ethanol to this solution，and 5 mL sodium hydroxide solution （2 mol/L） dropwise. Stir the reaction solution at room temperature for 5 minutes. Next，add 10 mL benzaldehyde and stir evenly. Keep this reaction mixture at room temperature for 1week.

（2）Finally，filter the above system，wash the filter cake with a small amount of ice water，dry and weigh it up. Calculate the the yield and measure the melting point.

### 2. Preparation of 1-phenyl-1,2-propanedione

（1） Equip the reaction experimental set-up as shown in Fig. 8-2. Add 2.12 g benzoin, 9.0 g ferric chloride hexahydrate and 5 mL water into the 100 mL three-neck round-bottom flask, and stir evenly. Add 10 mL glacial acetic acid, and heat the mixture to reflux and maintain for 1 h. Then, add 50 mL water is and continue heating and refluxing for 5 minutes.

（2） Cool the mixture to room temperature, and let the solid precipitate and filter. The filter cake is crude 1,2-diphenylacetone.

（3） Recrystallize the crude product with 12 mL ethanol, and filter, wash with a small amount of cold ethanol-ether solution, dry and weigh. Calculate the yield and measure the melting point.

### 3. Preparation of phenytoin

（1） Equip the reaction experimental set-up as shown in Fig. 8-2. Add 1 g 1-phenyl-1,2-propanedione, 0.57 g urea, 3.1 mL 15 % sodium hydroxide and 5 mL ethanol into the 100 mL three-neck round-bottom flask, heat the mixture to reflux for 2 h, and cool down to room temperature.

（2） Transfer the reaction solution to a beaker, add 37 mL distilled water, stir it evenly, put at room temperature for 15 minutes, filter, and adjust the pH= 4～5 with 15 % hydrochloric acid. Let the solid particles precipitate, filter and wash with a small amount of cold water. Once crude phenytoin is obtained, dry and weigh it up. Finally, calculate the yield and measure the melting point.

### 4. Preparation of phenytoin sodium

（1） Equip the reaction experimental set-up as shown in Fig. 8-2. Add 1 g phenytoin and 5 mL water into the 100 mL three-neck round-bottom flask and heat up to 40 ℃. Add 5 mL sodium hydroxide solution （15 %） slowly until the solid is completely dissolved. Next, add activated carbon and heat up the solution to 60 ℃ for 10 minutes. Filter the hot solution by vacuum filtration, stand it at room temperature for 20 minutes, and cool down with ice water. Solid paritcles will precipitate.

（2） Filter the solid precipitate and wash it with a small amount of ice water. Now, sodium phenytoin is obtained. Dry the product under infrared lamp. Weigh the pure product, measure the melting point and calculate the yield.

（3） Send the final product to the place where the guide teachers designated.

## V  Experimental Results

### 1. Yield

（1） Calculate the theoretical production of phenytoin sodium

$$\text{Benzaldehyde} \longrightarrow \text{Phenytoin sodium}$$
$$M_w = 106.12 \text{ g/mol} \longrightarrow M_w = 274.25 \text{ g/mol}$$
$$0.098 \text{ mol} \longrightarrow 0.049 \text{ mol}$$

Theoretical production$= 0.049 \text{ mol} \times 274.25 \text{ g/mol} = 13.44 \text{ g}$

(2) Calculate the percent yield of phenytoin sodium

$$\text{Yield} = \frac{\text{Practical production}}{\text{Theoretical production}} \times 100\% = \frac{(\quad\quad)}{13.44\text{ g}} \times 100\% = (\quad\quad)\%$$

## 2. Appearance and melting point of product

A. Appearance： _____ ；

B. m. p. ：

    Theoretical value：292～299 ℃

    Practical value： _____ .

## 3. Analysis of experimental results

_____

_____

_____

_____

_____

_____

_____ .

## Ⅵ Notes

1. Benzaldehyde used in benzoin preparation needs to be newly distilled.

2. When 1,2-diphenylethylene ketone is prepared，the reaction system should be in a mild boiling state.

3. The control of reaction temperature in each step is an important factor.

4. The whole reaction takes place in a sequence whereby the product of the one step will be used in the next step. So，the amount of reagent used should be calculated proportionally.

## Ⅶ Discussion Questions

1. Structurally，what is the mechanism of benzoin condensation catalyzed by Vitamin $B_1$？

2. Can benzoin be oxidized with concentrated nitric acid in the preparation of 1,2-diphenylethylene ketone?

3. Structurally，explain the reaction mechanism for the formation of phenytoin.

（By Yichao Zheng）

# 苯妥英钠的合成

## 背景知识

苯妥英钠（Phenytoin sodium），也称作大仑丁、地伦丁，为抗癫痫大发作首选药物，也用作抗心律失常药物，其化学结构式见图 8-1。

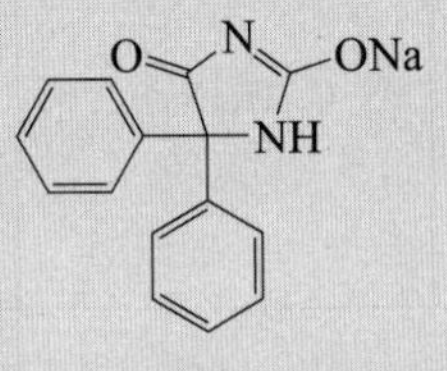

图 8-1　苯妥英钠化学结构式

苯妥英钠的作用靶标是电压门控钠离子通道（VGSC），选择 PDB：6AGF 为靶标蛋白进行分子模拟。**彩插 8** 显示了苯妥英钠和 VGSC 作用的结合模式图。**彩插 8A** 显示了苯妥英乙内酰脲上的 4 位氨基基团与残基 Tyr 1593 的苯环侧链形成阳离子-π 相互作用，苯妥英的两个苯环与周围疏水性残基 Phe 1601、Leu 443、Phe 805、Tyr 1593 等形成强疏水作用。此外，苯环与残基 Phe 1601 形成 π-π 堆积作用，并且苯妥英的两个苯环与酰胺基团其几乎成直角，与其他 S6 片段相互作用填充于孔腔，以阻滞 $Na^+$ 通道，减少 $Na^+$ 内流，从而使神经细胞膜稳定，并且阻止脑部病灶发生的异常电位活动向周围正常脑组织的扩散，起到抗癫痫作用。**彩插 8B** 显示苯妥英可以稳定地结合在 VGSC 的活性位点中心。

## Ⅰ　目的与要求

1. 掌握安息香缩合反应、氧化反应、重排反应的原理和操作要求。
2. 了解苯妥英钠与靶标的作用方式。

## Ⅱ　实验原理

### 1. 主要反应物和产物的物理常数

| 名称 | 结构式/CAS 号 | 分子式/分子量 | 沸点或熔点/℃ | 溶解度 |
|---|---|---|---|---|
| 苯甲醛 | CHO  100-52-7 | $C_7H_6O$  106.12 | b. p.  179 | 水：＜0.01 g/100 mL |
| 安息香 | OH O  119-53-9 | $C_{14}H_{12}O_2$  212.24 | m. p.  134～138 | 不溶于水，微溶于醚类，溶于醇 |
| 1,2-二苯乙二酮 | O O  579-07-7 | $C_9H_8O_2$  210.23 | m. p.  95～96 | 溶于乙醇、乙醚、丙酮、苯、氯仿等有机溶剂，不溶于水 |
| 苯妥英 | H O O NH  57-41-0 | $C_{15}H_{12}N_2O_2$  252.27 | m. p.  293～295 | 水：＜0.01 g/100 mL，溶于 DMSO |
| 苯妥英钠 | O N ONa NH  630-93-3 | $C_{15}H_{11}NaO_2$  274.25 | m. p.  292～299 | 易溶于水，溶于乙醇，不溶于氯仿 |
| 维生素 $B_1$ | $NH_2 \cdot HCl$ N $Cl^-$ N$^+$ S $H_3C$ $H_3C$ OH  67-03-8 | $C_{12}H_{16}N_4OS \cdot HCl$  337.27 | m. p.  245～250 | 极易溶于水，微溶于乙醇，不溶于乙醚、苯、氯仿和丙酮 |
| 六水合三氯化铁 | $FeCl_3 \cdot 6H_2O$  10025-77-1 | $FeCl_3 \cdot 6H_2O$  270.30 | m. p.  37 | 易溶于水 |
| 尿素 | $NH_2CONH_2$  57-13-6 | $CH_4N_2O$  60.06 | m. p.  132.7 | 溶于水、甲醇、甲醛、乙醇、液氨和醇，微溶于乙醚、氯仿、苯 |

## 2. 合成路线

苯甲醛 → 维生素 $B_1$ → 安息香 → $FeCl_3 \cdot 6H_2O$ → 1,2-二苯乙二酮

(1) $NH_2CONH_2$, NaOH
(2) HCl → 苯妥英 → NaOH → 苯妥英钠

苯甲醛在维生素 $B_1$ 催化下，发生安息香缩合生成安息香，然后，经氧化生成 1,2-二苯乙二酮，随后，在碱性条件下，与尿素缩合并经重排生成苯妥英，最后，经成盐反应得到苯妥英钠。

**安全提示**：苯甲醛对眼睛、呼吸道黏膜有一定的刺激作用。

## Ⅲ 实验装置和原料

### 1. 实验装置

反应实验装置如图 8-2 所示，主要由恒温磁力搅拌器、三颈烧瓶、球形冷凝管和温度计组成。

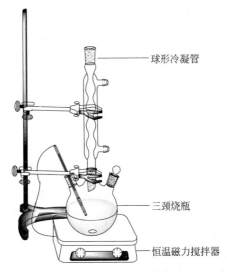

图 8-2 反应实验装置

### 2. 原料

| 合成步骤 | 原料 | | | |
|---|---|---|---|---|
| | 名称 | 用量 | 试剂级别 | 用途 |
| 安息香 | 苯甲醛 | 10 mL(0.098 mol) | 化学纯 | 反应物 |
| | 维生素 $B_1$ | 1.75 g(0.005 mol) | 化学纯(60 %) | 催化剂 |
| | 95 %乙醇 | 15 mL | — | 溶剂 |
| | 2 mol/L NaOH | 5 mL | — | 催化剂 |
| | 蒸馏水 | 适量 | — | 溶剂 |
| 1,2-二苯乙二酮 | 安息香 | 2.12 g (0.010 mol) | 自制 | 反应物 |
| | 六水合三氯化铁 | 9.0 g (0.033 mol) | 化学纯 | 氧化剂 |
| | 冰醋酸 | 10 mL | 化学纯 | 溶剂 |
| | 95 %乙醇 | 适量 | 化学纯 | 溶剂 |
| | 蒸馏水 | 适量 | — | 溶剂 |
| | 乙醚 | 适量 | 化学纯 | 溶剂 |

| 合成步骤 | 原料 | | | |
| --- | --- | --- | --- | --- |
| | 名称 | 用量 | 试剂级别 | 用途 |
| 苯妥英 | 1,2-二苯乙二酮 | 1 g | 自制 | 反应物 |
| | 尿素 | 0.57 g (0.0095 mol) | 化学纯 | 反应物 |
| | 15 %NaOH | 3.1 mL | 自制 | 催化剂 |
| | 95 %乙醇 | 5 mL | 化学纯 | 溶剂 |
| | 15 %盐酸 | 适量 | — | 中和反应 |
| | 蒸馏水 | 37 mL | — | 溶剂 |
| 苯妥英钠 | 苯妥英 | 1 g | 自制 | 反应物 |
| | 15 %氢氧化钠 | 5 mL | 自制 | 反应物 |
| | 活性炭 | 适量 | 化学纯 | 脱色剂 |
| | 蒸馏水 | 5 mL | — | 溶剂 |

## Ⅳ 实验操作

### 1. 安息香合成

（1）按图 8-2 所示搭建反应实验装置。在 50 mL 三颈烧瓶中，加入 1.75 g 维生素 $B_1$、4 mL 蒸馏水，搅拌溶解，向上述溶液中加入 15 mL 95 %乙醇，逐滴加入 5 mL 2 mol/L 氢氧化钠水溶液。滴加完毕，室温搅拌 5 min，加入 10 mL 苯甲醛，搅拌均匀后，室温放置 1 周。

（2）将以上体系抽滤，滤饼用少量冷水洗涤，烘干，称重，计算收率，测熔点。

### 2. 1,2-二苯乙二酮合成

（1）按图 8-2 所示搭建反应实验装置。在 100 mL 三颈烧瓶中，加入 2.12 g 安息香、9.0 g 六水合三氯化铁和 5 mL 水，搅拌均匀后，加入 10 mL 冰醋酸，升温至回流反应 1 h。然后加入 50 mL 水，继续加热回流 5 min。

（2）将反应体系冷却至室温，析出固体，抽滤，得到的滤饼即为 1,2-二苯乙酮粗品。

（3）把粗品用 12 mL 乙醇重结晶，抽滤，用少量冷的乙醇和乙醚混合溶液洗涤滤饼，干燥，称重，计算收率。测熔点。

### 3. 苯妥英合成

（1）按图 8-2 所示搭建反应实验装置。在 100 mL 三颈烧瓶中，加入 1 g 1,2-二苯乙二酮、0.57 g 尿素、3.1 mL 15 %氢氧化钠和 5 mL 95 %乙醇，升温至回流反应 2 h，降温至室温。

（2）将反应液转移至烧杯，加入 37 mL 蒸馏水，搅拌均匀，室温放置 15 min，抽滤。滤液用 15 %的盐酸调节 pH 值为 4～5。析出固体，抽滤，少量冷水洗涤滤饼，得到苯妥英粗品，干燥，称重，计算收率。测熔点。

### 4. 苯妥英钠合成

（1）按图 8-2 所示搭建反应实验装置。在 100 mL 三颈烧瓶中，加入 1 g 苯妥英和 5 mL 水，升温至 40 ℃，缓慢加入 15 %氢氧化钠水溶液 5 mL 直至固体完全溶解。加入活性炭，升温至 60 ℃并保温 10 min。热过滤，室温放置 20 min 后，冰水冷却。析出固体。

（2）过滤，少量冷水洗涤滤饼，真空干燥，得到苯妥英钠。称重，计算收率，测熔点。

（3）将产物送到指导教师指定的产品回收处。

## V 实验结果

**1. 收率**

（1）计算苯妥英钠的理论产量

$$苯甲醛————苯妥英钠$$

$$M_w=106.12 \text{ g/mol} ————M_w=274.25 \text{ g/mol}$$

$$0.098 \text{ mol} ————0.049 \text{ mol}$$

$$理论产量=0.049 \text{ mol}×274.25 \text{ g/mol}=13.44 \text{ g}$$

（2）计算苯妥英钠的收率

$$收率=\frac{产品实际产量}{产品理论产量}×100\%=\frac{(\quad\quad)}{13.44 \text{ g}}×100\%=(\quad\quad)\%$$

**2. 产品外观与熔点**

A. 外观：_____；

B. 熔点：

理论值：292～299 ℃

实测值：_____。

**3. 实验结果分析**

_____

_____

_____

_____

_____

_____.

## VI 注意事项

1. 安息香制备所用苯甲醛需要为新蒸馏过的。

2. 在制备 1,2-二苯乙二酮时，反应体系应为温和沸腾状态。

3. 各步骤反应温度控制是重要的因素。

4. 整个反应是接着上一步反应进行的，所用试剂的量需要按照比例计算后使用。

## VII 思考题

1. 用结构式表示维生素 $B_1$ 催化安息香缩合反应的机理。

2. 在制备 1,2-二苯乙二酮时，能用浓硝酸氧化安息香吗？

3. 用结构式表示合成苯妥英这一步反应的反应机理。

（郑一超）

# Experiment 9

# Synthesis of Neostigmine Bromide

## Background

Neostigmine bromide is a reversible anti-cholinesterase drug used for treatment of myasthenia gravis, intestinal paralysis and urinary retention after abdominal surgery. The chemical structure of neostigmine bromide is shown in Fig. 9-1.

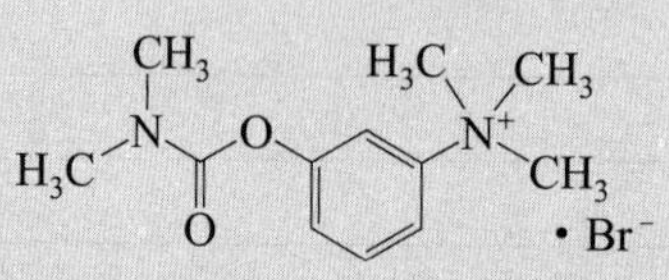

Fig. 9-1  Structure of Neostigmine Bromide

Acetylcholinesterase (AChE) is the target for neostigmine bromide and neostigmine bromide produce anticholinergic effect through inhibiting the hydrolysis of acetylcholine. Here, the crystal structure of AChE (PDB ID: 6F25) is used to predict the binding mode of neostigmine with the protein by molecular docking software. The mechanism of neostigmine and AChE was shown in Fig. 9-2 and **Color Diagram 9**. First, neostigmine binds to the active site of AChE to form a complex (**Color Diagram 9A**). The benzene group of neostigmine forms an aromatic-aromatic interaction with residue Trp 86, and the ester group is close to residue Ser 125 to prepare for further reaction. Next, the carbamoyl group of neostigmine binds to the hydroxyl group of Ser 125 at the active site of the AChE, and the ester bond is cleaved to form dimethylcarbamoyl- acetylcholinesterase (**Color Diagram 9B**) and 3-hydroxyphenyl- trimethylammonium. This causes the AChE to lose its ability to hydrolyze acetylcholine. The carbonyl group of dimethylcarbamoyl-acetylcholinesterase can be attacked by water molecule to reactivate the enzyme and separate dimethylcarbamic acid, and hence to restore the activity of AChE. However, the rate of hydrolysis of dimethylcarbamoyl-acetylcholinesterase is slower than the rate of AChE inhibition. So, the enzyme is inhibited for a longer period of time.

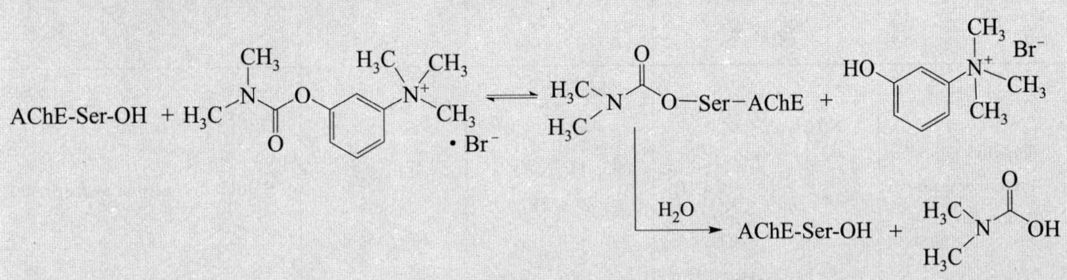

Fig. 9-2　Inhibition of acetylcholinesterase by bromoneostigmine

## I　Purposes and Requirements

1. To master the principle and operation requirements of $N$-alkylation reaction, esterification reaction principle and operation requirements.

2. To understand the interaction between neostigmine bromide and target.

## II　Principle of the Reaction

### 1. Physical data of the main reactants and product

| Name | Structure/CAS No. | Formula/M. Wt | b. p. or m. p. /℃ | Solubility |
|---|---|---|---|---|
| 3-Aminophenol | 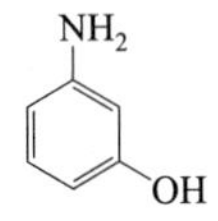 (structure) 591-27-5 | $C_6H_7NO$ 109.05 | m. p. 121 | Slightly soluble in water, ethanol and ether |
| Dimethyl sulfate | (structure) 77-78-1 | $C_2H_6O_4S$ 126.13 | b. p. 188 ℃ (Decompose) | Soluble in ethanol, ether, dioxane, acetone and aromatic hydrocarbons; Decomposition in water |
| 3-Dimethylamino- phenol | 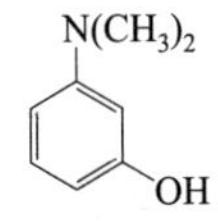 (structure) 99-07-0 | $C_8H_{11}NO$ 137.18 | m. p. 82~84 | Soluble in ethanol, ether, acetone, benzene, alkali and inorganic acid; almost insoluble in water |

| Name | Structure/CAS No. | Formula/M. Wt | b. p. or m. p. /℃ | Solubility |
|------|-------------------|---------------|-------------------|------------|
| Dimethylcarbamoyl chloride | $Cl-\overset{\overset{O}{\|}}{C}-N\overset{CH_3}{\underset{CH_3}{}}$ <br> 79-44-7 | $C_3H_6ClNO$ <br> 107. 54 | b. p. <br> 167～168 | Decompose in water; soluble in ether, benzene and carbon disulfide |
| 3-dimethylaminophenyl dimethylcarbamate (Neostigmine) | $N(CH_3)_2$ ... $O-\overset{\overset{O}{\|}}{C}-N\overset{CH_3}{\underset{CH_3}{}}$ <br> 16088-19-0 | $C_{11}H_{16}N_2O_2$ <br> 208. 26 | b. p. <br> 313. 6 | Soluble in acetone and ethanol |
| Neostigmine bromide | $N^+(CH_3)_3 \cdot Br^-$ ... $O-\overset{\overset{O}{\|}}{C}-N\overset{CH_3}{\underset{CH_3}{}}$ <br> 114-80-7 | $C_{12}H_{19}BrN_2O_2$ <br> 303. 2 | m. p. <br> 175～177 | Well soluble in water; soluble in ethanol and chloroform; insoluble in ether |
| Triethylamine | $N(CH_2CH_3)_3$ <br> 121-44-8 | $C_6H_{15}N$ <br> 101. 19 | b. p. <br> 89. 5 | — |
| Pyridine | (pyridine ring) <br> 110-86-1 | $C_5H_5N$ <br> 79. 1 | m. p. <br> 96～98 | Soluble in water and common organic solvents |
| Toluene | $CH_3$ (benzene ring) <br> 108-88-3 | $C_7H_8$ <br> 92. 14 | b. p. <br> 110 | Insoluble in water, soluble in most organic solvents such as benzene, alcohol and ether |
| Methyl bromide | $CH_3Br$ <br> 74-83-9 | $CH_3Br$ <br> 94. 94 | b. p. <br> 3. 6 | Insoluble in water; soluble in most organic solvents such as ethanol, ether, chloroform, benzene, etc. |

## 2. Synthetic route

3-Aminophenol         3-Dimethylaminophenol

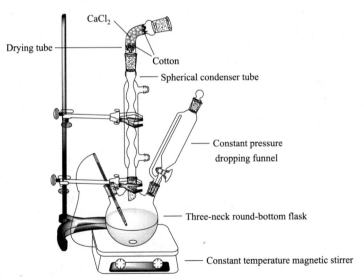

Neostigmine               Neostigmine bromide

3-Dimethylaminophenol is formed by $N$-alkylation of 3-aminophenol and dimethyl sulfate, which is subsequently esterified with $N,N$-dimethylcarbamoyl chloride to produce neostigmine. And then, neostigmine bromide was synthesized by quaternary ammoniation with methyl bromide.

**Safety Tips:** Dimethyl sulfate has strong irritating effect on eyes and upper respiratory tract, and strong corrosive effect on skin.

$N,N$-dimethylcarbamoyl chloride has strong irritation to eyes, skin, mucosa and respiratory tract. It should be used in the fume hood.

## Ⅲ Experimental Equipment and Raw Materials

### 1. Experimental equipment

Reaction experimental set-up （A）, Fig. 9-3, is composed from constant temperature magnetic stirrer, three-neck round-bottom flask, spherical condenser tube, thermometer, constant pressure dropping funnel and drying tube.

Fig. 9-3　Reaction experimental set-up （A）

Reaction experimental set-up （B）, Fig. 9-4, is composed from constant temperature magnetic stirrer, three-neck round-bottom flask, spherical condenser tube, gasing rubber tube and thermometer.

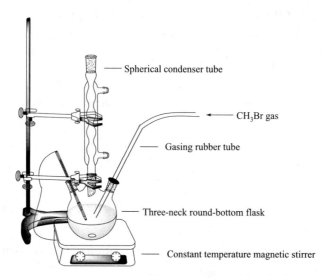

Spherical condenser tube

CH₃Br gas

Gasing rubber tube

Three-neck round-bottom flask

Constant temperature magnetic stirrer

Fig. 9-4 Reaction experimental set-up (B)

## 2. Raw materials

| Synthetic product | Raw materials | | | |
|---|---|---|---|---|
| | Name | Quantity | Quality | Use |
| 3-Dimethylaminophenol | 3-Aminophenol | 22 g (0.2 mol) | C. P. | Reactant |
| | Dimethyl sulfate | 38.8 mL (0.4 mol) | C. P. | Reactant |
| | Toluene | 50 mL | C. P. | Solvent |
| | Sodium carbonate | Proper amount | C. P. | Neutralization reaction |
| | Distilled water | Proper amount | — | Solvent |
| 3-dimethylaminophenyl dimethyl-carbamate (Neostigmine) | 3-Dimethylaminophenol | 13.7 g (0.1 mol) | Product prepared | Reactant |
| | Dimethylcarbamoyl chloride | 11.8 g (0.11 mol) | C. P. | Acylation reagent |
| | Triethylamine | 20.8 mL (0.15 mol) | C. P. | Acid-binding agent |
| | Pyridine | 1.6 mL (0.02 mol) | C. P. | Acid-binding agent |
| | Toluene | 100 mL | C. P. | Solvent |
| | NaOH | Proper amount | C. P. | Neutralization reaction |
| | Distilled water | Proper amount | — | Solvent |
| | Silica Gel for Chromatography | 5 g | C. P. | Adsorption impurity |
| | Anhydrous sodium sulfate | proper amount | C. P. | Dehydrant |
| Neostigmine bromide | Neostigmine | 10.4 g (0.05 mol) | Product prepared | Reactant |
| | Methyl bromide | 4.1 mL (0.075 mol) | C. P. | Reactant |
| | Acetone | 20 mL | C. P. | Solvent |
| | Absolute ethanol | 30 mL | C. P. | Solvent |
| | Activated carbon | 0.5 g | C. P. | Discolouring agent |

# Ⅳ Operations

### 1. Preparation of 3-dimethylaminophenol

（1）Equip the reaction experimental set-up （A） as Fig. 9-3. Add 22 g 3-aminophenol and 50 mL toluene into the 250 mL three-neck round-bottom flask, and dissolve it completely by stirring. Next, add 38. 8 mL dimethyl sulfate （treated with anhydrous sodium carbonate to pH＝5） dropwise within 30 minutes. Heat up the the solution to 75 ℃ for 3 h and cool down to room temperature.

（2）Separate the organic layer and adjust the pH to 9 with sodium carbonate solution. Separate the organic layer again and remove toluene by rotating evaporation. Distill the residues by vacuum distillation at 138～150 ℃/10 mmHg and collect the fraction. 3-Dimethyl-aminophenol is obtained when the fraction is frozen. Dry the product under infrared lamp and weigh it up. Calculate the yield and measure the melting point.

### 2. Preparation of neostigmine

（1）Equip the reaction experimental set-up （B） as shown in Fig. 9-3. Add 13. 7 g 3-Dimethylaminophenol, 20. 8 mL triethylamine, 1. 6 mL pyridine and 100 mL toluene into the 250 mL three-neck round-bottom flask and stir it evenly. Add 7. 1 g $N$, $N$-dimethylcarbamoyl chloride dropwise at room temperature and heat to 45～50 ℃ for 3 h.

（2）Cool the reaction solution to room temperature, add 100 mL distilled water and stir evenly. Separate the organic layer, wash it with 10 ％ sodium hydroxide solution, and add anhydrous sodium sulfate to dry overnight.

（3）Remove the sodium sulfate by filtration. Add 5 g silica gel to the organic layer and stir it evenly. Remove the silica gel by filtration. Rotate the filtrate to remove the solvent. The residue is neostigmine. Dry the product under infrared lamp and weigh it up. Calculate the yield and measure the melting point.

### 3. Preparation of neostigmine bromide

（1）Equip the reaction experimental set-up as shown in Fig. 9-4. Add 10. 4 g neostigmine and 20 mL acetone into the 100 mL three-neck round-bottom flask and cool it to 5 ℃. Add 4. 1 mL methane bromide and stored at room temperature for 3 days. Crystals will precipitate.

（2）The crude neostigmine bromide is obtained by filtration.

（3）Dissolve the crude product in anhydrous ethanol （30 mL）, then reflux with 0. 5 g activated carbon for 5 minutes. Filter the hot solution and cool it to room temperature. Precipitate the solids and filter. Wash the filter cake is with a small amount of cold ethanol to obtain the pure bromo-neostigmine.

（4）Dry the product under infrared lamp and weigh it up. Calculate the yield and measure the melting point.

（5）Send the finished product to the place where the guide teachers designated.

# Ⅴ Experimental Results

### 1. Yield

（1）Calculate the theoretical production of neostigmine bromide

$$3\text{-Aminophenol} \longrightarrow \text{Neostigmine bromide}$$

$$M_w = 109.05 \text{ g/mol} \longrightarrow M_w = 303.2 \text{ g/mol}$$

$$0.2 \text{ mol} \longrightarrow 0.2 \text{ mol}$$

$$\text{Theoretical production} = 0.2 \text{ mol} \times 303.2 \text{ g/mol} = 60.64 \text{ g}$$

(2) Calculate the percent yield of neostigmine bromide

$$\text{Yield} = \frac{\text{Practical production}}{\text{Theoretical production}} \times 100\% = \frac{(\quad)}{60.64 \text{ g}} \times 100\% = (\quad)\%$$

## 2. Appearance and melting point of product

Physical Identification

A. Appearance: _____ ;

B. m. p. :

  Theoretical value: 175～177 ℃

  Practical value: _____ .

## 3. Analysis of experimental results

_____

_____

_____

_____

_____

_____

_____ .

## Ⅵ Notes

1. The synthetic step of 3-dimethylaminophenol is anhydrous reaction. The reagents and instruments used need to be dried before use.

2. When neostigmine bromide is refined, if the product does not precipitate at room temperature, it should be placed in ice bath at 0 ℃.

3. The control of reaction temperature in each step is an important factor.

4. The whole reaction takes place in a sequence whereby the product of the one step will be used in the next step. So, the amount of reagent used should be calculated proportionally.

## Ⅶ Discussion Questions

1. Structurally, what substances can be used to replace triethylamine in the esterification reaction to produce neostigmine?

2. Structurally, explain the reaction mechanism for the formation of neostigmine.

(By Wen Li，Hongmin Liu)

# 实验九

# 溴新斯的明的合成

## 背景知识

溴新斯的明（Neostigmine bromide），是一种可逆性抗胆碱酯酶药，用于重症肌无力、腹部术后的肠麻痹和尿潴留等症，其化学结构式见图 9-1。

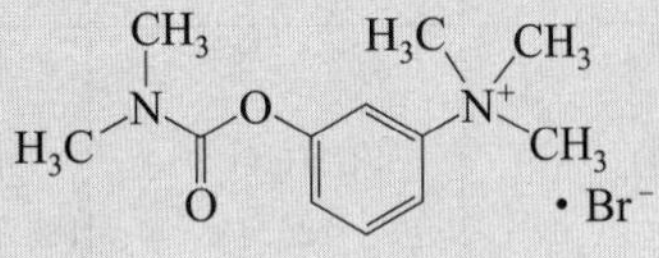

图 9-1 溴新斯的明化学结构式

溴新斯的明的作用靶标是乙酰胆碱酯酶，通过抑制乙酰胆碱的水解发挥抗胆碱作用，选择 PDB：6F25 为靶标蛋白进行分子模拟。采用分子对接软件 MOE，预测新斯的明与乙酰胆碱酯酶的结合模式，其作用机制如图 9-2 和**彩插 9** 所示。首先，新斯的明结合到乙酰胆碱酯酶的活性位点，生成复合物（**彩插 9A**），其中，新斯的明的苯环与 Trp 86 形成芳环-芳环相互作用，脂基靠近 Ser 125，为下一步反应做准备；随后，新斯的明的氨基甲酰基与酶活性中心的 Ser 125 羟基结合，酯键断裂，生成二甲胺基甲酰化乙酰胆碱酯酶（**彩插 9B**）和 3-羟基苯基三甲胺，从而失去酶对乙酰胆碱的水解能力，发挥抗胆碱酯酶作用。直到水分子攻击二甲胺基甲酰化胆碱酯酶的羰基，重新激活酶，可分离出二甲胺基甲酸，胆碱酯酶活性得以恢复。二甲胺基甲酰化胆碱酯酶的水解速度较乙酰化胆碱酯酶的水解速度慢，故酶被抑制的时间较长。

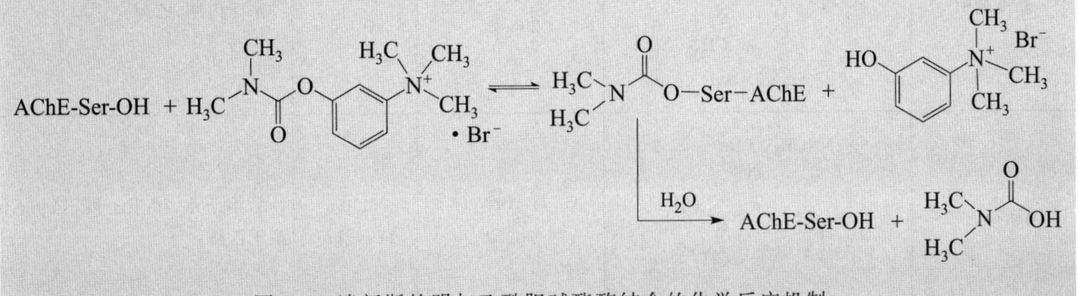

图 9-2 溴新斯的明与乙酰胆碱酯酶结合的化学反应机制

# Ⅰ 目的与要求

1. 掌握 N-烷基化反应、酯化反应原理、操作要求。
2. 了解溴新斯的明与靶标作用方式。

# Ⅱ 实验原理

## 1. 主要反应物和产物的物理常数

| 名称 | 结构式/CAS 号 | 分子式/分子量 | 沸点或熔点/℃ | 溶解度 |
|---|---|---|---|---|
| 间氨基苯酚 | 591-27-5 | $C_6H_7NO$<br>109.05 | m. p.<br>121 | 微溶于水,溶于醇、醚 |
| 硫酸二甲酯 | 77-78-1 | $C_2H_6O_4S$<br>126.13 | b. p.<br>188 ℃(分解) | 溶于乙醇、乙醚、二氧六环、丙酮和芳香烃类,遇水分解 |
| 间二甲氨基苯酚 | 99-07-0 | $C_8H_{11}NO$<br>137.18 | m. p.<br>82~84 | 溶于乙醇、乙醚、丙酮、苯、碱和无机酸,几乎不溶于水 |
| N,N-二甲氨基甲酰氯 | 79-44-7 | $C_3H_6ClNO$<br>107.54 | b. p.<br>167~168 | 遇水分解,溶于乙醚、苯和二硫化碳 |
| 新斯的明 | 16088-19-0 | $C_{11}H_{16}N_2O_2$<br>208.26 | b. p.<br>313.6 | 溶于丙酮,乙醇 |
| 溴新斯的明 | 114-80-7 | $C_{12}H_{19}BrN_2O_2$<br>303.2 | m. p.<br>175~177 | 易溶于水,溶于乙醇、氯仿,不溶于乙醚 |

| 名称 | 结构式/CAS 号 | 分子式/分子量 | 沸点或熔点/℃ | 溶解度 |
|---|---|---|---|---|
| 三乙胺 | $N(CH_2CH_3)_3$<br>121-44-8 | $C_6H_{15}N$<br>101.19 | b. p.<br>89.5 | — |
| 吡啶 | 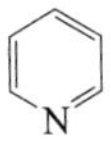 <br>110-86-1 | $C_5H_5N$<br>79.1 | m. p.<br>96~98 | 可溶于水和常用有机溶剂 |
| 甲苯 | 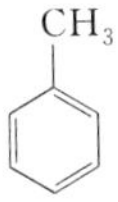 <br>108-88-3 | $C_7H_8$<br>92.14 | b. p.<br>110 | 不溶于水,可混溶于苯、醇、醚等多数有机溶剂 |
| 溴甲烷 | $CH_3Br$<br>74-83-9 | $CH_3Br$<br>94.94 | b. p.<br>3.6 | 不溶于水,溶于乙醇、乙醚、氯仿、苯等多数有机溶剂 |

### 2. 合成路线

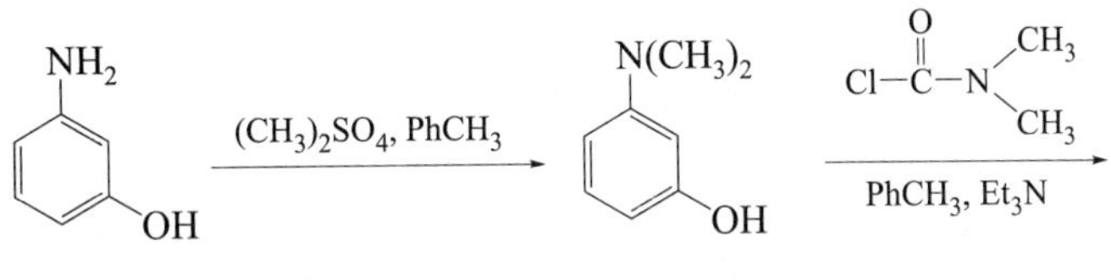

3-氨基苯酚          3-二甲氨基苯酚

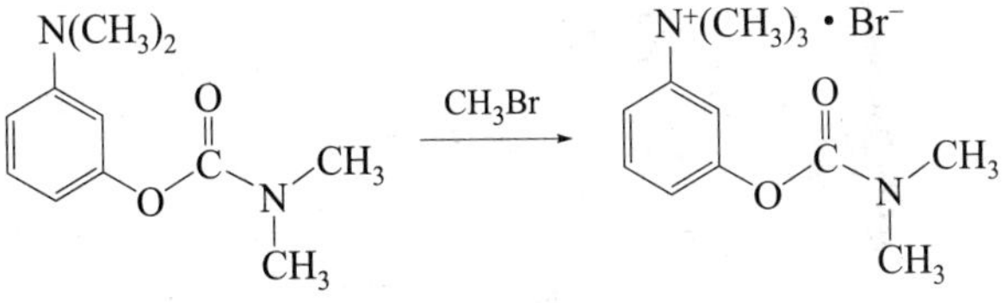

新斯的明          溴新斯的明

3-氨基苯酚与硫酸二甲酯发生 $N$-烷基化反应生成 3-二甲氨基苯酚,然后与 $N,N$-二甲氨基甲酰氯发生酯化反应生成新斯的明,随后,与溴甲烷成季铵盐得到溴新斯的明。

**安全提示**:硫酸二甲酯对眼睛、上呼吸道有强烈刺激作用,对皮肤有强腐蚀作用。

$N,N$-二甲氨基甲酰氯对眼睛、皮肤黏膜和呼吸道有强烈的刺激作用。故使用该试剂时应在通风橱中使用。

## Ⅲ 实验装置和原料

### 1. 实验装置

反应实验装置(A)如图 9-3 所示,主要用由恒温磁力搅拌器、三颈烧瓶、球形冷凝管、温度计、滴液漏斗和干燥管组成。

反应实验装置(B)如图 9-4 所示,主要由恒温磁力搅拌器、三颈烧瓶、球形冷凝管、导气管和温度计组成。

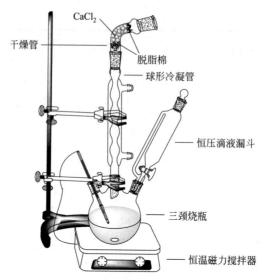

图 9-3  反应实验装置（A）

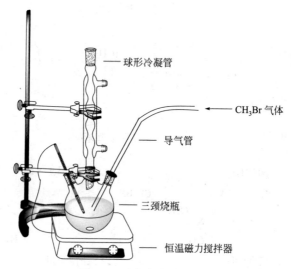

图 9-4  反应实验装置（B）

## 2. 原料

| 合成产物 | 原料 | | | |
|---|---|---|---|---|
| | 名称 | 用量 | 试剂级别 | 用途 |
| 3-二甲氨基苯酚 | 3-氨基苯酚 | 22 g(0.2 mol) | 化学纯 | 反应物 |
| | 硫酸二甲酯 | 38.8 mL(0.4 mol) | 化学纯 | 反应物 |
| | 甲苯 | 50 mL | 化学纯 | 溶剂 |
| | 碳酸钠 | 适量 | 化学纯 | 中和酸 |
| | 蒸馏水 | 适量 | — | 溶剂 |
| 新斯的明 | 3-二甲氨基苯酚 | 13.7 g(0.1 mol) | 自制 | 反应物 |
| | $N,N$-二甲氨基甲酰氯 | 7.1 g(0.11 mol) | 化学纯 | 酰化试剂 |
| | 三乙胺 | 20.8 mL(0.15 mol) | 化学纯 | 缚酸剂 |

| 合成产物 | 原料 | | | |
|---|---|---|---|---|
| | 名称 | 用量 | 试剂级别 | 用途 |
| 新斯的明 | 吡啶 | 1.6 mL(0.02 mol) | 化学纯 | 缚酸剂 |
| | 甲苯 | 100 mL | 化学纯 | 溶剂 |
| | 氢氧化钠 | 适量 | 化学纯 | 中和酸 |
| | 蒸馏水 | 适量 | — | 溶剂 |
| | 层析用硅胶 | 5 g | 化学纯 | 吸附杂质 |
| | 无水硫酸钠 | 适量 | 化学纯 | 干燥除水 |
| 溴新斯的明 | 新斯的明 | 10.4 g(0.05 mol) | 自制 | 反应物 |
| | 溴甲烷 | 4.1 mL(0.075 mol) | 化学纯 | 反应物 |
| | 丙酮 | 20 mL | 化学纯 | 溶剂 |
| | 无水乙醇 | 30 mL | 化学纯 | 溶剂 |
| | 活性炭 | 0.5 g | 化学纯 | 脱色剂 |

## Ⅳ 实验操作

### 1. 间二甲氨基苯酚合成

（1）按图 9-3 所示搭建实验装置（A）。在 250 mL 三颈烧瓶中，加入 22 g 3-氨基苯酚和 50 mL 甲苯，搅拌溶解，在 30 min 内逐滴加入 38.8 mL 硫酸二甲酯（用无水碳酸钠处理至 pH 值为 5）。滴加完毕，升温至 75 ℃反应 3 h。冷却至室温。

（2）分取有机层，加碳酸钠水溶液调节 pH＝9，再次分取有机层，旋转蒸发除去甲苯，残留物减压蒸馏，收集 138～150 ℃/10 mmHg 的馏分，固化后得到 3-二甲氨基苯酚，称重，计算收率，测熔点。

### 2. 新斯的明合成

（1）按图 9-3 所示搭建实验装置（A）。在 250 mL 三颈烧瓶中，加入 13.7 g 3-二甲氨基苯酚、20.8 mL 三乙胺、1.6 mL 吡啶和 100 mL 甲苯，搅拌均匀后，室温滴加 7.1 g $N,N$-二甲氨基甲酰氯，升温至 45～50 ℃反应 3 h。

（2）反应体系冷却至室温，加入蒸馏水 100 mL，搅拌均匀后，分取有机层，10 ％氢氧化钠溶液洗涤，加入无水硫酸钠干燥过夜。

（3）过滤除去硫酸钠，有机层加入层析用硅胶 5 g 搅拌均匀，过滤，滤液旋转除去溶剂，残留物为新斯的明。称重，计算收率。

### 3. 溴新斯的明合成

（1）按图 9-4 所示搭建实验装置（B）。在 100 mL 三颈烧瓶中，加入 10.4 g 新斯的明和 20 mL 丙酮，冷却至 5 ℃后，通入 4.1 mL 溴甲烷，室温放置 3 天。析出晶体。

（2）过滤，得到溴新斯的明粗品。

（3）将粗品用 30 mL 无水乙醇加热溶解，加入活性炭回流 5 min，过滤，冷却至室温，析出固体，抽滤，少量冷乙醇洗涤滤饼，得到溴新斯的明精制品。

（4）烘干纯品，称重，计算收率，测熔点。

（5）将产物送到指导教师指定的产品回收处。

## Ⅴ 实验结果

### 1. 收率
（1）计算溴新斯的明的理论产量

$$3\text{-}氨基苯酚 \text{————} 溴新斯的明$$
$$M_w=109.05 \text{ g/mol} \text{————} M_w=303.2 \text{ g/mol}$$
$$0.2 \text{ mol} \text{————} 0.2 \text{ mol}$$
$$理论产量=0.2 \text{ mol}\times303.2 \text{ g/mol}=60.64 \text{ g}$$

（2）计算溴新斯的明的收率

$$收率=\frac{产品实际产量}{产品理论产量}\times100\% = \frac{(\qquad)}{60.64 \text{ g}}\times100\% = (\qquad)\%$$

### 2. 产品外观与熔点
A. 外观：＿＿＿＿＿＿＿＿＿＿＿＿＿＿＿＿＿＿＿；

B. 熔点：

　　理论值：175～177 ℃

　　实测值：＿＿＿＿＿＿＿＿＿＿＿＿＿＿＿＿＿。

### 3. 实验结果分析

＿＿＿＿＿＿＿＿＿＿＿＿＿＿＿＿＿＿＿＿＿＿＿＿＿＿＿＿＿＿＿＿＿＿＿＿＿＿

＿＿＿＿＿＿＿＿＿＿＿＿＿＿＿＿＿＿＿＿＿＿＿＿＿＿＿＿＿＿＿＿＿＿＿＿＿＿

＿＿＿＿＿＿＿＿＿＿＿＿＿＿＿＿＿＿＿＿＿＿＿＿＿＿＿＿＿＿＿＿＿＿＿＿＿＿

＿＿＿＿＿＿＿＿＿＿＿＿＿＿＿＿＿＿＿＿＿＿＿＿＿＿＿＿＿＿＿＿＿＿＿＿＿＿

＿＿＿＿＿＿＿＿＿＿＿＿＿＿＿＿＿＿＿＿＿＿＿＿＿＿＿＿＿＿＿＿＿＿＿＿＿＿

＿＿＿＿＿＿＿＿＿＿＿＿＿＿＿＿＿＿＿＿＿＿＿＿＿＿＿＿＿＿＿＿＿＿＿＿＿．

## Ⅵ 注意事项

1. 3-二甲氨基苯酚合成步骤为无水反应，所用试剂和仪器需要干燥后使用。

2. 在溴新斯的明精制时，若室温不析出产品，冰浴 0 ℃放置。

3. 各步骤反应温度控制是重要的因素。

4. 整个反应是接着上一步反应进行的，所用试剂的量需要按照比例计算后使用。

## Ⅶ 思考题

1. 用结构式表示，酯化反应生成新斯的明时，可用什么物质取代三乙胺？

2. 用结构式表示，生成新斯的明这一步反应的反应机理。

（李雯　刘宏民）

# Experiment 10

# Synthesis of Dyclonine Hydrochloride

## Background

Dyclonine hydrochloride, also named dacronin, is an aminone local anesthetic developed by Swiss Astrazeneca Company. It has been used in China since 2002. This product has the advantages of strong mucosal penetration, rapid response and lasting effect. Clinically, it is used for analgesia of burns and abrasions, and for preparation before endoscopy such as laryngoscope, tracheoscope and cystoscopy. The chemical structure of dyclonine hydrochloride is shown in Fig. 10-1.

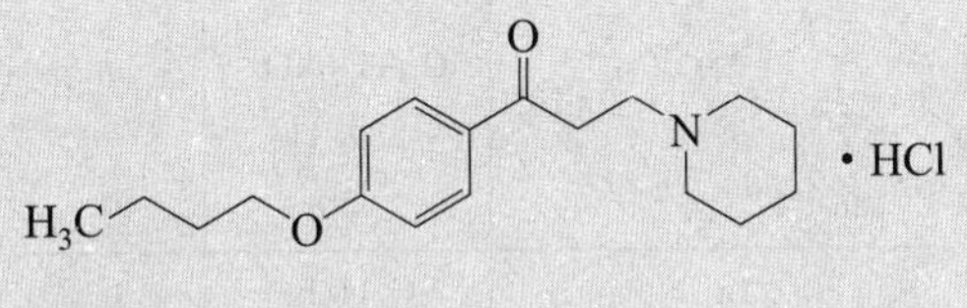

Fig. 10-1　Structure of Dyclonine Hydrochloride

Voltage-gated sodium channels (VGSC) are the target for local anesthetics and PDB: 6AGF was selected as the target protein. The crystal structures of dyclonine and VGSC are shown in **Color Diagram 10**. The binding pattern of phenytoin is shown in **Color Diagram 10A**, the butoxyphenyl group forms strong hydrophobic interactions with the surrounding hydrophobic residues Phe 1284, Phe 1586 and Tyr 1593, so that dyclonine could stably occupy the inner pore of the VGSC to prevent $Na^+$ penetration and block membrane depolarization, thereby exerting local anesthesia effect. **Color Diagram 10B** clearly shows that dyclonine can stably bind to the active site of VGSC.

# I Purposes and Requirements

1. To master the principle and operation requirements of $O$-alkylation reaction, Mannich reaction.

2. To understand the application of phase transfer catalytic reaction in drug synthesis.

3. To understand the interaction between dyclonine hydrochloride and target.

# II Principle of the Reaction

## 1. Physical data of the main reactants and product

| Name | Structure/CAS No. | Formula/ M. Wt | b. p. or m. p. /℃ | Solubility |
|---|---|---|---|---|
| $p$-Hydroxyaceto-phenone | 99-93-4 | $C_8H_8O_2$ 136. 15 | m. p. $107\sim111$ | Well soluble in hot water, methanol, ethanol, ether, acetone, benzene; insoluble in petroleum ether; it can dissolve in 100 phr of water at 22 ℃ and 14 phr of water at 100 ℃ |
| 4-Butoxyaceto-phenone | 5736-89-0 | $C_{12}H_{16}O_2$ 192. 25 | m. p. $25\sim27$ | — |
| Dyclonine hydro-chloride | 586-60-7 | $C_{18}H_{27}NO_2$ 289. 41 | m. p. $175\sim176$ | Well soluble in water; soluble in chloroform, acetone and methanol |
| 1-Bromobutane | 109-65-9 | $C_4H_9Br$ 137. 03 | b. p. 101. 6 | — |
| Tetrabutylammo-nium bromide | $(n\text{-}C_4H_9)_4N^+\cdot Br^-$ 1643-19-2 | $C_{16}H_{36}BrN$ 322. 37 | m. p. $100\sim106$ | Well soluble in water, ethanol, ether and acetone; slightly soluble in benzene |
| Potassium carbon-ate | $K_2CO_3$ 584-08-7 | $K_2CO_3$ 138. 21 | m. p. 891 | Well soluble in water |
| Paraformaldehyde | $(HCHO)_n$ 30525-89-4 | $(CH_2O)_n(30)_n$ | m. p. $120\sim170$ | Soluble in dilute alkali and acid solution; more soluble in hot water; insoluble in ethanol and ether |
| Piperidine hydro-chloride | 6091-44-7 | $C_5H_{12}ClN$ 121. 61 | m. p. $245\sim248$ | Well soluble in water and ethanol |
| Dichloromethane | $CH_2Cl_2$ 75-09-2 | $CH_2Cl_2$ 84. 93 | b. p. 40 | Soluble in organic solvents such as ethyl acetate and ethanol; insoluble in water |

| Name | Structure/CAS No. | Formula/ M. Wt | b. p. or m. p. /°C | Solubility |
|------|-------------------|----------------|---------------------|------------|
| Hydrochloric acid | HCl<br>7647-01-0 | HCl<br>36. 5 | b. p. 48(38 % solutinon) | Aqueous solution |
| Etanol | $CH_3CH_2OH$<br>64-17-5 | $C_2H_6O$<br>46. 07 | b. p.<br>78 | Miscible with water and organic solvents such as ether, chloroform, glycerol, methanol,etc. |
| Diethyl ether | $(CH_2CH_3)_2O$<br>60-29-7 | $C_4H_{10}O$<br>74. 12 | b. p.<br>34. 6 | Soluble in low-carbon ethanols, benzene, chloroform, petroleum ethers and oils; slightly soluble in water |
| Sodium sulfate | $Na_2SO_4$<br>7757-82-6 | $Na_2SO_4$<br>142. 04 | m. p.<br>884 | Soluble in water |

\* $n\text{-}C_4H_9 = CH_3CH_2CH_2CH_2$

## 2. Synthetic route

p-Hydroxyacetophenone → 4-Butoxyacetophenone

Dyclonine hydrochloride

p-Butoxyacetophenone is obtained by O-alkylation from p-hydroxyacetophenone and n-bromobutane. And then, p-butoxyacetophenone, polyformaldehyde and piperidine hydrochloride will undergo mannich condensation to form dyclonine hydrochloride.

**Safety Tips**: Mixture of diethyl ether vapor and air is explosive gas, which is easy to burn and explode in open fire and high heat. Explosive peroxides can be produced after long exposure to air. Pay attention to ventilate when using.

## Ⅲ Experimental Equipment and Raw Materials

### 1. Experimental equipment

Reaction experimental set-up (A), Fig. 10-2, is composed from four-neck round-bottom flask, spherical condenser tube, constant temperature magnetic stirrer, thermometer and cosstant pressure dropping funnel.

Reaction experimental set-up (B), Fig. 10-3, is composed from three-neck round-bottom flask, spherical condenser tube, constant temperature magnetic stirrer and thermometer.

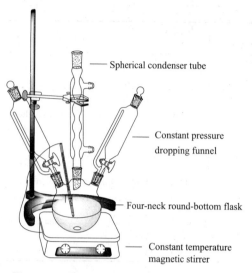

Fig. 10-2　Reaction experimental set-up（A）

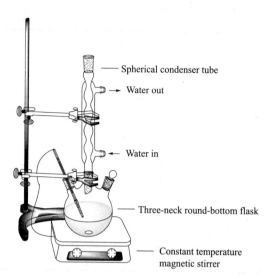

Fig. 10-3　Reaction experimental set-up（B）

## 2. Raw materials

| Synthetic product | Raw materials | | | |
| --- | --- | --- | --- | --- |
| | Name | Quantity | Quality | Use |
| 4-Butoxyaceto-phenone | $p$-Hydroxyacetophenone | 6. 8 g (0. 05 mol) | C. P. | Reactant |
| | 1-Bromobutane | 8. 3 mL (0. 077 mol) | C. P. | Reactant |
| | Potassium carbonate | 6. 9 g (0. 05 mol) | C. P. | Reactant |
| | Tetrabutylammonium bromide | 0. 4 g (0. 00125 mol) | C. P. | Phase transfer catalyst |
| | Dichloromethane | 60 mL | C. P. | Solvent |
| | Distilled water | 60 mL | — | Solvent |
| | Anhydrous sodium sulfate | 3 g | C. P. | Dehydrant |
| Dyclonine hydrochloride | 4-Butoxyacetophenone | 8. 7 g (0. 045 mol) | Product prepared | Reactant |
| | Paraformaldehyde | 2. 7 g (0. 09 mol) | C. P. | Reactant |
| | Piperidine hydrochloride | 7. 3 g (0. 06 mol) | C. P. | Reactant |
| | Concentrated hydrochloric acid | 0. 6 mL | C. P. | Catalytic agent |
| | Ethanol | 85 mL | C. P. | Solvent |
| | Diethyl ether | 40 mL | C. P. | Solvent |
| | Distilled water | Proper amount | — | Solvent |

## Ⅳ　Operations

### 1. Preparation of 4-butoxyacetophenone

（1）Equip the reaction experimental set-up（A）as shown in Fig. 10-2. Add 0. 4 g tetra-butylammonium bromide，10 mL dichloromethane and 10 mL distilled water into the 250 mL four-neck round-bottom flask，and heat up the reaction mixture to 40 ℃ while stirring until dissolved completely.

(2) Dissolve 6. 9 g potassium carbonate in 50 mL water in a 100 mL beaker and then add 6. 8 g $p$-hydroxyacetone. Stir the solution until dissolved completely.

(3) Dissolve 8. 3 mL $n$-Bromobutane (8. 3 mL) in 50 mL dichloromethane in a 100 mL beaker. Stir the solution evenly.

(4) Add the solution of $p$-hydroxyacetone and the solution of $n$-bromobutane prepared in step 3 and 4 dropwise to the flask at the simultaneously, and stir vigorously. Keep the reaction going on for further 2 h at 40 ℃. The mixture is then cooled to room temperature.

(5) Separate the organic layer and extract the aqueous layer with 20 mL dichloromethane. Pool the organic layers together, and add anhydrous sodium sulfate and put overnight. Remove sodium sulfate by filtration and dry the filtrate by evaporation to obtain oily substances. Weigh the oil and calculate the yield.

### 2. Preparation of neostigmine

(1) Equip the reaction experimental set-up (B) as shown in Fig. 10-3. Add 8. 7 g $p$-butoxy acetophenone, 2. 7 g polyformaldehyde, 7. 3 g piperidine hydrochloride, 0. 6 mL concentrated hydrochloric acid and 85 mL ethanol into the 250 mL three-neck round-bottom flask, heat to reflux and maintain for 3 h, then cool down to room temperature.

(2) Add 50 mL water into the reaction solution, the mixture is extracted by ether and the water layer is separated.

(3) The water layer is heated to 60 ℃, stirred to clarify, cooled to room temperature. Solid is precipitated and filtered. The crude dyclonine hydrochloride is obtained.

(4) The crude dyclonine hydrochloride is recrystallized with ethanol-water (1 : 9) mixed solvent. The ratio of solute to solvent is crude product : ethanol-water＝1 g : 8 mg. The mixture is heated and dissolved, cooled to room temperature. The solid is precipitated and filtered. The filter cake is washed with a small amount of cold ethanol to obtain the pure dacronin hydrochloride.

(5) Dry the pure product under infrared lamp. Weigh the pure product, calculate the yield and measure the melting point.

(6) Send the final product to the place where the guide teachers designated.

## V Experimental Results

### 1. Yield

(1) Calculate the theoretical production of dyclonine hydrochliorid

$p$-Hydroxyacetophenone ———— Dyclonine hydrochloride

$M_w$＝136. 15 g/mol ————$M_w$＝289. 41 g/mol

0. 05 mol ————0. 05 mol

Theoretical production＝0. 05 mol×289. 41 g/mol＝14. 47 g

(2) Caculate the percent yield of dyclonine hydrochloride

$$\text{Yield}=\frac{\text{Practical production}}{\text{Theoretical production}}\times 100\ \%=\frac{(\qquad)}{14.47\text{ g}}\times 100\ \%=(\qquad)\%$$

## 2. Appearance and melting point of product

A. Appearance：_____ ；

B. m. p. ：

    Theoretical value：175～176 ℃

    Practical value：_____ .

## 3. Analysis of experimental results

_____

_____

_____

_____

_____

_____

_____ .

# Ⅵ  Notes

1. O-alkylation is a phase transfer reaction system. Because it is a multi-phase system, sufficient stirring is the key factor to improve the conversion of the reaction.

2. Usually，in order to promote reaction，Mannich reaction needs to use oil-water separator to remove water from the reaction system. After times exploration，the preparation of dyclonine hydrochloride can still obtain a higher yield when using ethanol reflux method without oil-water separator. The reaction operation is more simple.

3. The whole reaction takes place in a sequence whereby the product of the one step will be used in the next step. So，the amount of reagent used should be calculated proportionally.

# Ⅶ  Discussion Questions

1. Structurally，why dose p-hydroxyacetophenone dissolve in potassium carbonate aqueous solution?

2. Structurally，explain the reaction mechanism of Mannich condensation to dyclonine hydrochlorid.

(By Qiurong Zhang)

# 实验十

# 盐酸达克罗宁的合成

## 背景知识

盐酸达克罗宁（Dyclonine hydrochloride）是瑞士 Astrazeneca 公司开发的氨基酮类局部麻醉药物，2002 年在我国开始应用。该品具有黏膜穿透力强、显效快、作用持久的优点，临床常用于火伤、擦伤的镇痛，以及喉镜、气管镜、膀胱镜等内窥镜检查前的准备，其化学结构式见图 10-1。

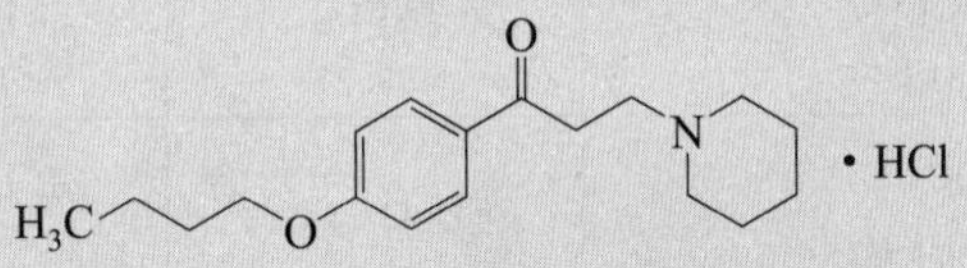

图 10-1　盐酸达克罗宁的化学结构式

盐酸达克罗宁作用靶标是电压门控 Na$^+$ 通道（VGSC），为钠通道阻滞剂，选择 PDB：6AGF 为靶标蛋白进行分子模拟。**彩插 10** 显示了盐酸达克罗宁和 VGSC 作用的作用模式图。如**彩插 10A** 显示，达克罗宁的正丁氧基苯基与 Phe 1284、Phe 1586、Tyr 1593 等疏水性残基形成较强的疏水作用，使得达克罗宁稳定地占据 VGSC 中心，以阻止 Na$^+$ 渗透，使传导阻滞，产生局部麻醉作用。**彩插 10B** 显示达克罗宁可以稳定地结合在 VGSC 的局麻药结合位点。

## Ⅰ　目的与要求

1. 掌握 O-烷基化反应、Mannich 反应的原理和操作要求。
2. 了解相转移催化反应在药物合成中的应用。
3. 了解盐酸达克罗宁与靶标的作用方式。

## Ⅱ　实验原理

### 1. 主要反应物和产物的物理常数

| 名称 | 结构式/CAS 号 | 分子式/分子量 | 沸点或熔点/℃ | 溶解度 |
|------|------------|------------|------------|--------|
| 对羟基苯乙酮 | ![结构式] 99-93-4 | $C_8H_8O_2$ 136.15 | m. p. 107~111 | 易溶于热水、甲醇、乙醇、乙醚、丙酮、苯;难溶于石油醚;22 ℃时可溶于100 份水中,100℃时可溶于 14 份水中 |
| 对正丁氧基苯乙酮 | $n$-$C_4H_9^*$ 结构式 5736-89-0 | $C_{12}H_{16}O_2$ 192.25 | m. p. 25~27 | — |
| 盐酸达克罗宁 | $n$-$C_4H_9O$ 结构式 ·HCl 586-60-7 | $C_{18}H_{27}NO_2$ 289.41 | m. p. 175~176 | 易溶于水;溶于氯仿、丙酮、甲醇 |
| 正溴丁烷 | $n$-$C_4H_9Br$ 109-65-9 | $C_4H_9Br$ 137.03 | b. p. 101.6 | — |
| 溴化四丁基铵 | $(n$-$C_4H_9)_4N^+ \cdot Br^-$ 1643-19-2 | $C_{16}H_{36}BrN$ 322.37 | m. p. 100~106 | 易溶于水、乙醇、乙醚和丙酮;微溶于苯 |
| 碳酸钾 | $K_2CO_3$ 584-08-7 | $K_2CO_3$ 138.21 | m. p. 891 | 易溶于水 |
| 多聚甲醛 | $(HCHO)_n$ 30525-89-4 | $(CH_2O)_n (30)_n$ | m. p. 120~170 | 溶于稀碱和稀酸溶液;较易溶于热水;不溶于醇和醚 |
| 哌啶盐酸盐 | NH·HCl 6091-44-7 | $C_5H_{12}ClN$ 121.61 | m. p. 245~248 | 易溶于水和乙醇 |
| 二氯甲烷 | $CH_2Cl_2$ 75-09-2 | $CH_2Cl_2$ 84.93 | b. p. 40 | 与乙酸乙酯、乙醇等有机溶剂互溶,不溶于水 |
| 盐酸 | HCl 7647-01-0 | HCl 36.5 | b. p. 48(38 %溶液) | 水溶液 |
| 乙醇 | $CH_3CH_2OH$ 64-17-5 | $C_2H_6O$ 46.07 | b. p. 78 | 与水混溶;可混溶于乙醚、氯仿、甘油、甲醇等多数有机溶剂 |
| 乙醚 | $CH_3CH_2OCH_2CH_3$ 60-29-7 | $C_4H_{10}O$ 74.12 | b. p. 34.6 | 溶于低碳醇、苯、氯仿、石油醚和油类;微溶于水 |
| 无水硫酸钠 | $Na_2SO_4$ 7757-82-6 | $Na_2SO_4$ 142.04 | m. p. 884 | 溶于水 |

\* $n$-$C_4H_9 = CH_3CH_2CH_2CH_2$

**2. 合成路线**

对羟基苯乙酮 $\xrightarrow[(n\text{-}C_4H_9)_4N^+ \cdot Br^-]{n\text{-}C_4H_9Br/K_2CO_3}$ 对正丁氧基苯乙酮

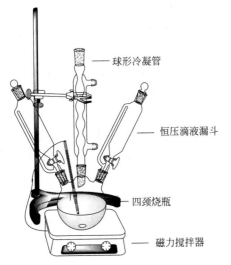

$$\xrightarrow{\text{(HCHO)}_n,\ \text{NH·HCl}} \quad \text{盐酸达克罗宁}$$

对羟基苯乙酮与正溴丁烷发生 $O$-烷基化反应生成对正丁氧基苯乙酮，然后与多聚甲醛和盐酸哌啶发生 Mannich 缩合生成盐酸达克罗宁。

**安全提示**：乙醚蒸气与空气可形成爆炸性混合物，遇明火、高热极易燃烧爆炸。在空气中久置后能生成有爆炸性的过氧化物。使用时应注意通风。

## Ⅲ 实验装置和原料

### 1. 实验装置

反应实验装置（A）如图 10-2 所示，主要由四颈烧瓶、球形冷凝管、磁力搅拌器、恒压滴液漏斗和温度计组成。

反应实验装置（B）如图 10-3 所示，主要由由三颈烧瓶、球形冷凝管、磁力搅拌器和温度计组成。

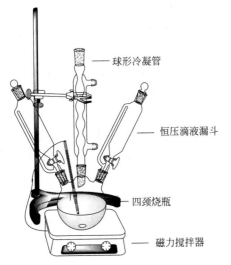

图 10-2　反应实验装置（A）

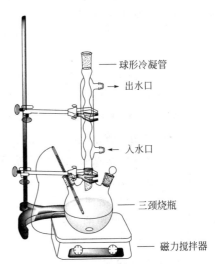

图 10-3　反应实验装置（B）

### 2. 原料

| 合成产物 | 原料 | | | |
|---|---|---|---|---|
| | 名称 | 用量 | 试剂级别 | 用途 |
| 对正丁氧基苯乙酮 | 对羟基苯乙酮 | 6.8 g(0.05 mol) | 化学纯 | 反应物 |
| | 正溴丁烷 | 8.3 mL(0.077 mol) | 化学纯 | 反应物 |
| | 碳酸钾 | 6.9 g(0.05 mol) | 化学纯 | 反应物 |
| | 溴化四丁基铵 | 0.4 g(0.00125 mol) | 化学纯 | 相转移催化剂 |
| | 二氯甲烷 | 60 mL | 化学纯 | 溶剂 |
| | 蒸馏水 | 60 mL | — | 溶剂 |

| 合成产物 | 原料 | | | |
|---|---|---|---|---|
| | 名称 | 用量 | 试剂级别 | 用途 |
| 对正丁氧基苯乙酮 | 无水硫酸钠 | 3 g | 化学纯 | 除水剂 |
| 盐酸达克罗宁 | 对正丁氧基苯乙酮 | 8.7 g(0.045 mol) | 自制 | 反应物 |
| | 多聚甲醛 | 2.7 g(0.09 mol) | 化学纯 | 反应物 |
| | 哌啶盐酸盐 | 7.3 g(0.06 mol) | 化学纯 | 反应物 |
| | 浓盐酸 | 0.6 mL | 化学纯 | 催化剂 |
| | 乙醇 | 85 mL | 化学纯 | 溶剂 |
| | 乙醚 | 40 mL | 化学纯 | 溶剂 |
| | 蒸馏水 | 适量 | — | 溶剂 |

## Ⅳ 实验操作

### 1. 对正丁氧基苯乙酮合成

（1）按图 10-2 所示搭建反应实验装置（A）。在 250 mL 四颈烧瓶中，加入 0.4 g 溴化四丁基铵、10 mL 二氯甲烷和 10 mL 蒸馏水，搅拌溶解，升温至 40 ℃。

（2）在 100 mL 烧杯，将 6.9 g 碳酸钾溶于 50 mL 水溶液中，加入 6.8 g 对羟基苯乙酮，搅拌溶解。

（3）在 100 mL 烧杯，将 8.3 mL 正溴丁烷加入 50 mL 二氯甲烷中，搅拌均匀。

（4）将配制好的对羟基苯乙酮水溶液和正溴丁烷溶液同时滴加入反应瓶中，剧烈搅拌，加料完毕，保持 40 ℃继续反应 2 h。冷却至室温。

（5）分取有机相，将水相用 20 mL 二氯甲烷提取，合并有机相和二氯甲烷提取液，加入无水硫酸钠，过夜。抽滤除去硫酸钠，滤液旋转蒸发至干，得到油状物。称重，计算收率。

### 2. 盐酸达克罗宁合成

（1）按图 10-3 所示搭建反应实验装置（B）。在 250 mL 三颈烧瓶中，加入 8.7 g 对正丁氧基苯乙酮、2.7 g 多聚甲醛、7.3 g 哌啶盐酸盐、0.6 mL 盐酸和 85 mL 乙醇，加热至回流，反应 3 h。冷却至室温。

（2）向反应体系中加入 50 mL 水，用乙醚萃取，分取水相。

（3）水相加热至 60 ℃搅拌至澄清，冷却至室温，析出晶体，过滤，得到盐酸达克罗宁粗品。

（4）粗品用乙醇-水（1∶9）混合溶剂重结晶，溶质与溶剂的用量比例为粗品∶乙醇-水＝1 g∶8 mL。加热溶解后，冷却至室温，析出固体，抽滤，少量冷乙醇洗涤滤饼，得到盐酸达克罗宁精制品。

（5）烘干纯品，称重，计算收率，测熔点。

（6）将产物送到指导教师指定的产品回收处。

## Ⅴ 实验结果

### 1. 收率

（1）计算盐酸达克罗宁的理论产量

対羟基苯乙酮—————盐酸达克罗宁
$M_w = 136.15 \text{ g/mol}$ —————$M_w = 289.41 \text{ g/mol}$
0.05 mol —————0.05 mol

理论产量 $= 0.05 \text{ mol} \times 289.41 \text{ g/mol} = 14.47 \text{ g}$

（2）计算盐酸达克罗宁的收率

$$收率 = \frac{产品实际产量}{产品理论产量} \times 100\% = \frac{(\quad\quad)}{14.47 \text{ g}} \times 100\% = (\quad\quad)\%$$

**2. 产品外观与熔点**

A. 外观：＿＿＿＿＿＿＿＿＿＿＿＿＿＿＿＿＿＿＿；

B. 熔点：

理论值：175～176 ℃；

实测值：＿＿＿＿＿＿＿＿＿＿＿＿＿＿＿＿＿。

**3. 实验结果分析**

＿＿＿＿＿＿＿＿＿＿＿＿＿＿＿＿＿＿＿＿＿＿＿＿＿＿＿＿＿＿＿＿＿＿
＿＿＿＿＿＿＿＿＿＿＿＿＿＿＿＿＿＿＿＿＿＿＿＿＿＿＿＿＿＿＿＿＿＿
＿＿＿＿＿＿＿＿＿＿＿＿＿＿＿＿＿＿＿＿＿＿＿＿＿＿＿＿＿＿＿＿＿＿
＿＿＿＿＿＿＿＿＿＿＿＿＿＿＿＿＿＿＿＿＿＿＿＿＿＿＿＿＿＿＿＿＿＿
＿＿＿＿＿＿＿＿＿＿＿＿＿＿＿＿＿＿＿＿＿＿＿＿＿＿＿＿＿＿＿＿＿＿
＿＿＿＿＿＿＿＿＿＿＿＿＿＿＿＿＿＿＿＿＿＿＿＿＿＿＿＿＿＿＿＿＿＿
＿＿＿＿＿＿＿＿＿＿＿＿＿＿＿＿＿＿＿＿＿＿＿＿＿＿＿＿＿＿＿＿＿＿
＿＿＿＿＿＿＿＿＿＿＿＿＿＿＿＿＿＿＿＿＿＿＿＿＿＿＿＿＿＿＿＿＿＿．

# Ⅵ 注意事项

1. O-烷基化反应为相转移反应体系，由于该反应体系是多相体系，充分的搅拌是提高反应转化率的关键因素。

2. 通常情况下，Mannich 反应需要采用油水分离器将水从反应体系中除去以促进反应进行，经反复探索，盐酸达克罗宁的制备可采用乙醇回流的方法，不必采用分水装置，依然可以得到较高收率，反应操作更为简便。

3. 整个反应是接着上一步反应进行的，所用试剂的量需要按照比例计算后使用。

# Ⅶ 思考题

1. 用结构式表示，为什么对羟基苯乙酮能溶于碳酸钾水溶液？

2. 用结构式表示，经 Mannich 缩合生成盐酸达克罗宁的反应机理。

（张秋荣）

# Appendix 1   Experimental Report Template

## Experiment 2   Synthesis of Aspirin

### I   Objectives of this Experiment

1. To master the acetylation reaction and its use on structural modification of drug substances.

2. To master the anhydrous operation method; and the use of coloration reaction on the end-poinl determination of organic synthesis.

3. To understand the interaction between aspirin and target.

### II   Principle of the Reaction

$$\text{Salicylic acid} + \text{Acetic anhydride} \xrightarrow{H_2SO_4} \text{Aspirin} + CH_3COOH$$

Salicylic acid          Acetic anhydride                Aspirin          Acetic acid

### III   Experimental Equipment and Raw Materials

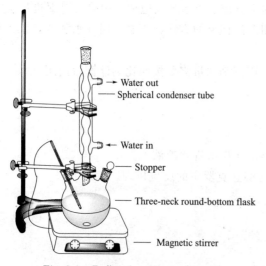

Fig. 2-1   Reflux experimental set-up

→ Water out
— Spherical condenser tube
← Water in
— Stopper
— Three-neck round-bottom flask
— Magnetic stirrer

1. Experimental equipment

Reflux experimental set-up (Fig. 2-1) is composed from three-neck round-bottom flask , spherical condenser tube, magnetic stirrer, thermometer.

Buchner funnel for vacuum filtration (Fig. 2-2) is composed from filter flask, Buchner funnel, filter paper and vacuum pump.

2. Raw materials

Different raw materials will be used in this experiment. They are:

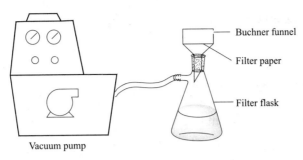

Fig. 2-2　Vacuum filtration experimental set-up

| Name | Quantity | Quality | Use |
|---|---|---|---|
| Salicyclic acid | 8. 3 g (0. 06 mol) | C. P. | Principle reactive |
| Acetic anhydride | 15 mL (0. 159 mol) | C. P. | Acetylating agent |
| Sulfuric acid | 0. 4 mL (5 drops) | C. P. | Catalyst |
| Ethanol | 12 mL | 95 % | Solvent for recryst |
| $FeCl_3$ reagent | 1 drop | — | End point measurement |
| $Na_2CO_3$ | 10 mL | — | Hydrolysing agent |
| $H_2SO_4$ diluted | 10 mL | — | Neutralizing agent |
| Active carbon(Charcoal) | 0. 5 g | — | Decolorizing substance |

## Ⅳ　Operations

Creat a data table to record the necessary quantitative information for this lab, as well as your observations of what occurred.

| No. | Experimental operation | Experimental phenomena |
|---|---|---|
| 1 | Take 15 mL of acetic acid anhydride and 5 drops of concentrated sulfuric acid and place them in 100 mL three-neck round-bottom flask. Assemble the reflux experimental set-up (as Fig. 2-1). Agitate gently; in parallel, raising the temperature at $55 \sim 60$ ℃ on the steam bath. | It took five minutes to rise temperature from room to $55 \sim 60$ ℃. |
| 2 | Add 8. 3 g of salicylic acid crystals to the reaction mixture; dissolve them and keep at $55 \sim 60$ ℃. Then, white crystals aspirin will appear. | It took 15 minutes to dissolve, and a colorless clarifying solution was obtained. |
| 3 | ... | ... |
| 4 | ... | ... |
| 5 | ... | ... |

# Ⅴ  Experimental Results

## 1. Yield

$$\text{Yield} = \frac{\text{Practical production}}{\text{Theoretical production}} \times 100\% = \frac{(\qquad)}{10.81\text{ g}} \times 100\% = (\qquad)\%$$

## 2. Appearance and melting point of product

A. Appearance：_____；

B. m. p. ：

　　Theoretical value：135～138 ℃

　　Practical value：_____。

## 3. Analysis of experimental results

The yield of aspirin in this experiment is 60%. Although the yield is considerable，there are still possibilities for further improvement，such as：（1）washing flasks with a small amount of solvent to collect product when the reaction solution is transferred；（2）thermal filtration is faster during recrystallization operation；and（3）the amount of recrystallization solvent should be controlled as much as possible in just dissolving solids. The melting range of the product is short and the value is in accordance with the theoretical value. It shows that the content of the product is high. The structure of the product can be further confirmed by NMR，MS，IR and elemental analysis. The content of the product can be further confirmed by high performance solution chromatography（HPLC）.

# Ⅵ  Discussion Questions

1. Structurally，why dose/might our room smell like vinegar during this experiment?

2. Structurally，why salicyclic and acetylsalicylic acid considered acids?

Salicylic acid

Aspirin[2- (acetyloxy) -benzoic acid]

# 附录一 实验报告模板

## 实验二 阿司匹林的合成

### I 实验目的

1.掌握酯化反应原理和其在药物结构改造中的应用。
2.掌握无水反应操作；掌握颜色反应在反应终点判断方面的应用。
3.了解阿司匹林的作用机制。

### II 实验原理

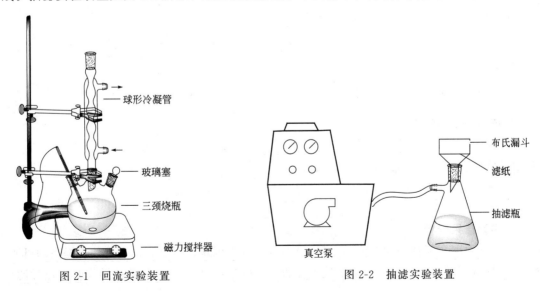

水杨酸       醋酸酐       阿司匹林       醋酸

### III 实验装置和原料

**1. 实验装置**

回流实验装置如图 2-1 所示，主要由三颈烧瓶、球形冷凝管、磁力搅拌器、温度计组成。抽滤实验装置如图 2-2 所示，主要由抽滤瓶、布氏漏斗、滤纸和真空泵组成。

图 2-1 回流实验装置             图 2-2 抽滤实验装置

**2. 原料**

| 名称 | 用量 | 试剂级别 | 用途 |
|---|---|---|---|
| 水杨酸 | 8.3 g(0.06 mol) | 化学纯 | 反应物 |
| 醋酸酐 | 15 mL(0.159 mol) | 化学纯 | 酰化试剂 |
| 浓硫酸 | 0.4 mL(5 drops) | 化学纯 | 催化剂 |
| 乙醇 | 12 mL | 95 % | 重结晶溶剂 |
| $FeCl_3$ 试液 | 1drop | — | 终点指示剂 |
| $Na_2CO_3$ | 10 mL | — | 水解剂 |
| 稀 $H_2SO_4$ | 10 mL | — | 中和试剂 |
| 活性炭 | 0.5 g | — | 脱色剂 |

## Ⅳ 实验过程

合成和分离 （列表，详实记录实验现象）

| 步骤 | 实验操作 | 实验现象 |
|---|---|---|
| 1 | 如图 2-1 所示搭建反应实验装置。在 100 mL 三颈烧瓶中，加入 15 mL 醋酸酐和 5 滴浓硫酸，在搅拌状态下，升温至 55～60 ℃。 | 从室温升高到 55～60 ℃用了 5 min。 |
| 2 | 在以上体系中，加入 8.3 g 水杨酸晶体，搅拌溶解保持温度 55～60 ℃，可观察到白色晶体逐渐溶解。 | 搅拌溶解用了 15 min，得到无色澄清溶液。 |
| 3 | … | … |
| 4 | … | … |
| 5 | … | … |

## Ⅴ 结果

**1. 收率**

$$收率 = \frac{产品实际产量}{产品理论产量} \times 100\% = \frac{(\qquad)}{10.8\ g} \times 100\% = (\qquad)\%$$

**2. 产品外观与熔点**

A. 外观：＿＿＿＿＿＿＿＿＿＿＿＿＿＿＿＿＿＿＿＿＿；

B. 熔点：

理论值：135～138 ℃

实测值：＿＿＿＿＿＿＿＿＿＿＿＿＿＿＿＿＿。

**3. 实验结果分析**

本实验中阿司匹林的收率为 60 %，虽然收率较为可观，但是，仍有进一步提高的可能，如（1）反应液转移时，用少量溶剂洗涤烧瓶，以收集产品；（2）重结晶操作时，热过滤更为迅速；（3）重结晶溶剂的用量尽可能控制在能恰好溶解固体等。所测得的产品的熔程较短，数值与理论值相符，说明产品含量较高，进一步确证产物结构，可采用核磁共振（NMR）、质谱（MS）、红外光谱（IR）和元素分析仪进行分析，进一步确证产物含量，可采用高效液相色谱（HPLC）进行分析。

## Ⅵ 思考题

1.用结构式表示，为什么在反应过程中室内会有醋酸的味道？

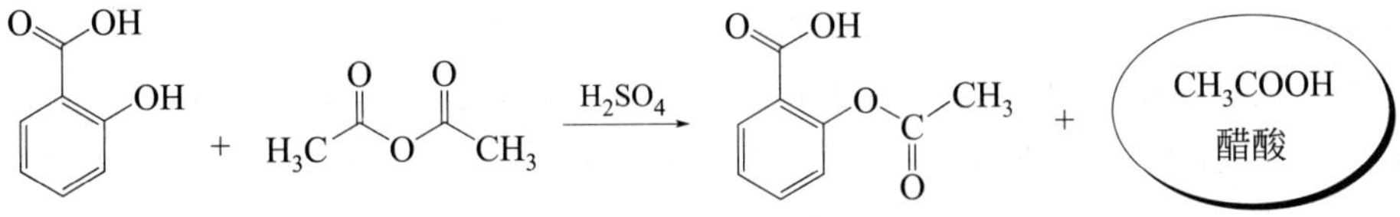

2.用结构式表示，为什么水杨酸和阿司匹林是酸性物质？

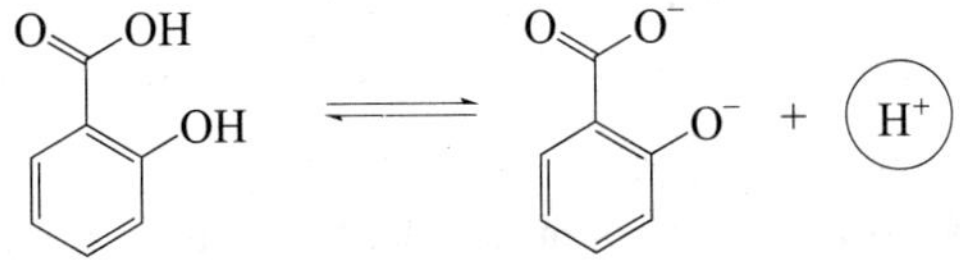

水杨酸

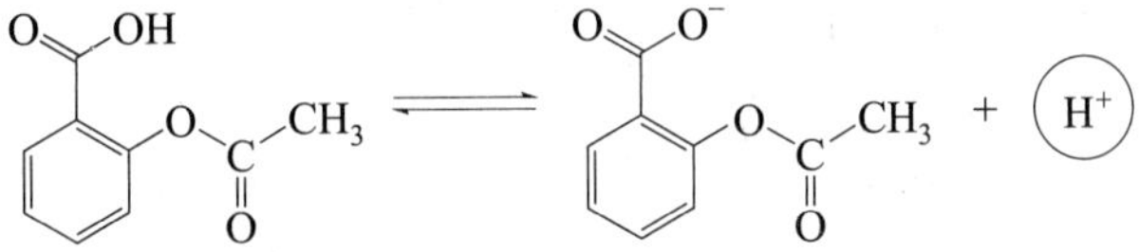

阿司匹林(2-乙酰氧基苯甲酸)

# Appendix 2 Reference Answer for the Discussion Questions

**Experiment 1**

**1. Why the activated carbon can not be added to the boiling solution when it used as a decolorizing agent?**

**Answer:** When the solution is boiling, adding activated carbon is easy to cause the serious bumping. Therefore, when the activated carbon is added, the solution must be slightly cold.

**2. What are the commonly used recrystallization solvents?**

**Answer:** Water, chloroform, acetone, ethyl acetate, ethanol, methanol, etc.

**Experiment 2**

**1. Structurally, why dose/might our room smell like vinegar during this experiment?**

**Answer:**

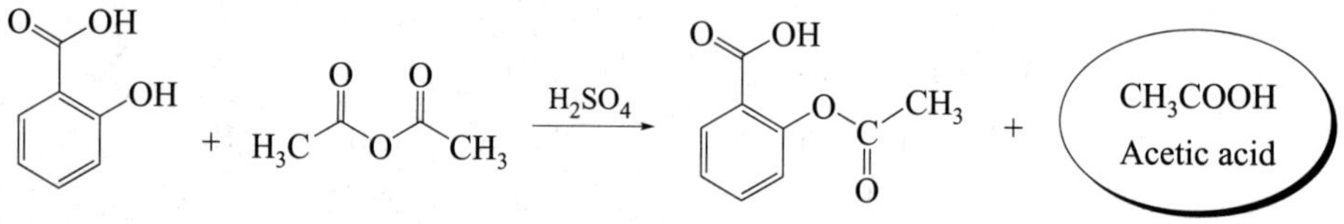

**2. Structurally, why salicyclic and acetylsalicylic acid are considered asacids?**

**Answer:**

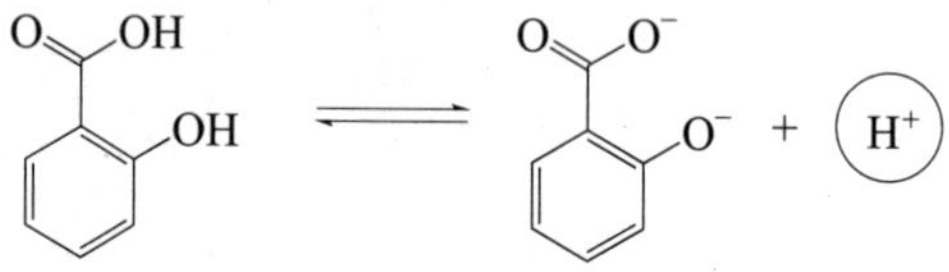

Salicylic acid

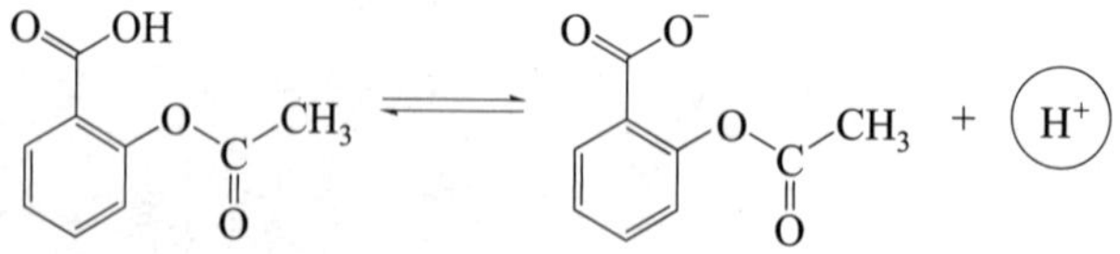

Aspirin[2- (acetyloxy) -benzoic acid]

**Experiment 3**

**1. Can acetic acid be used as an acylating agent in this preparation?**

**Answer:** Using acetic acid as the acylating agent, the reaction time is long, many side product may also be produced, and the quality of the product is poor.

**2. What are the common acylating agents?**

**Answer:** The common acylating agents and the order of their activity is:

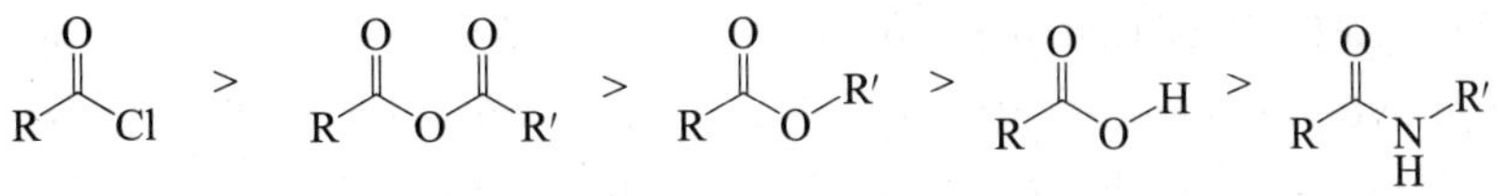

## 3. What are the common impurities of paracetamol?

**Answer:** The common impurities of paracetamol are:

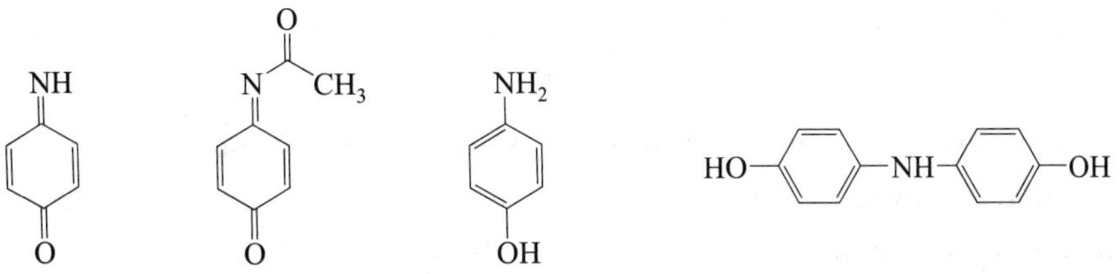

## Experiment 4

**1. Why benorilate cannot be prepared directly from aspirin and paracetamol?**

**Answer:** The electron density on the phenolic hydroxyl of paracetamol is low because of the conjugating of the phenolic hydroxyl to the benzene ring, which causes the weak nucleophilicity; the electron density of the phenolic oxygen atom is increased and beneficial to nucleophilic reaction after being salified. In addition, salifying can also avoid generating hydrogen chloride which can cause the hydrolysis of the resulting ester bond.

**2. What are the common reagents for the preparation of carboxylic chloride from carboxylic acid?**

**Answer:** $SOCl_2$, $(COCl)_2$, $PCl_3$, $PCl_5$.

**3. Why should some pyridine be added in the preparation of acetyl salicylic chloride? What will happen if pyridine is added in excess?**

**Answer:** Pyridine can catalize the reaction and eccelerate the reaction speed. The amout of pyridine used as a catalyst should not be excessive, otherwise the quality of the product will be affected.

## Experiment 5

**1. During the reaction, what are the solids precipitated at pH=7 and pH=5? What is the insoluble solid in 10 % hydrochloric acid?**

**Answer:** The precipitated solid at pH=7 are the sulfanilamide which don't participate in the reaction; the precipitated solid at pH=5 is sulfacetamide; the insoluble material in 10 % hydrochloric acid is sulfonamidacetyl which cannot be salted out because of the absence of free aromatic primary amino groups in the structure.

**2. During the reaction, it is very important to adjust pH between 12 and 13, and what will happen if alkaline is too strong or too weak?**

**Answer:** If alkaline is too strong, the product will be hydrolyzed, so will genetate more sulfonamides but less sulfonamide diacetyl. In contrast, sulfonamidacetyl can't hydrolyze easily, so it will genetate more sulfonamidacetyl but less sulfonamide.

## Experiment 6

**1. When the oxidation reaction is completed, on which chemical properties did the separation of p-nitrobenzoic acid from the mixture depends?**

**Answer**: Due to the fact that $p$-nitrobenzoic acid is insoluble in water, soluble impurity in water was removed by vacuum filtration in the oxidation reaction. When the solution was adjusted to alkalinity, $p$-nitrobenzoic acid was transferred to sodium $p$-nitrobenzoic. Sodium $p$-nitrobenzoic was soluble in water. Insoluble impurity in water was removed by vacuum filtration. When the solution was adjusted to acid, sodium $p$-nitrobenzoic was retransferred to $p$-nitrobenzoic acid. The solid was got by vacuum filtration to gain final product $p$-nitrobenzoic acid.

**2. Why water-free operation is needed in the esterification reaction?**

**Answer**: Esterification reaction is reversible reaction. If water goes into the reaction system, the material will not be consumed enough. The yield will be reduced.

**Experiment 7**

**1. Structurally, what substances can be used instead of sodium hydride?**

**Answer**: $CH_3ONa$, $CH_3CH_2ONa$, etc.

**2. Structurally, what substances can be used instead of Lewis acid $ZnCl_2$?**

**Answer**: $AlCl_3$, $BF_3 \cdot EtOEt$, $FeCl_3$, etc.

**3. Structurally, what substances can be used instead of 3-methyl-l-butanol?**

**Answer**: $CH_3CH_2CH_2CH_2CH_2OH$, $(CH_3)_3COH$, $CH_3CH_2CH_2CH_2OH$, etc.

**4. Structurally, what substances are the by-product of piperazine reaction of 6-fluoro in the condensation reaction of piperazine?**

**Answer**:

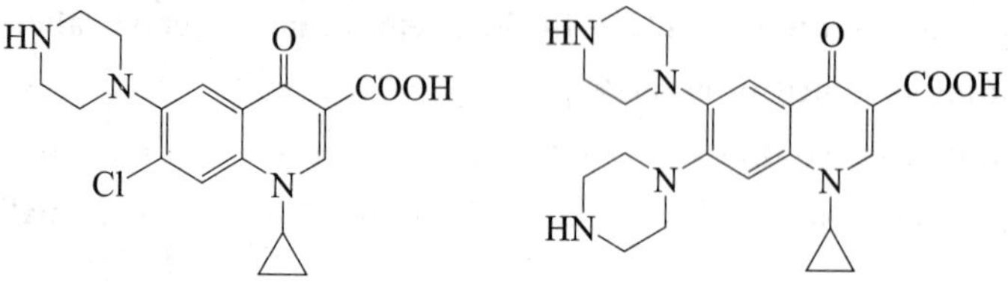

**Experiment 8**

**1. Structurally, what is the mechanism of benzoin condensation catalyzed by Vitamin $B_1$?**

**Answer**:

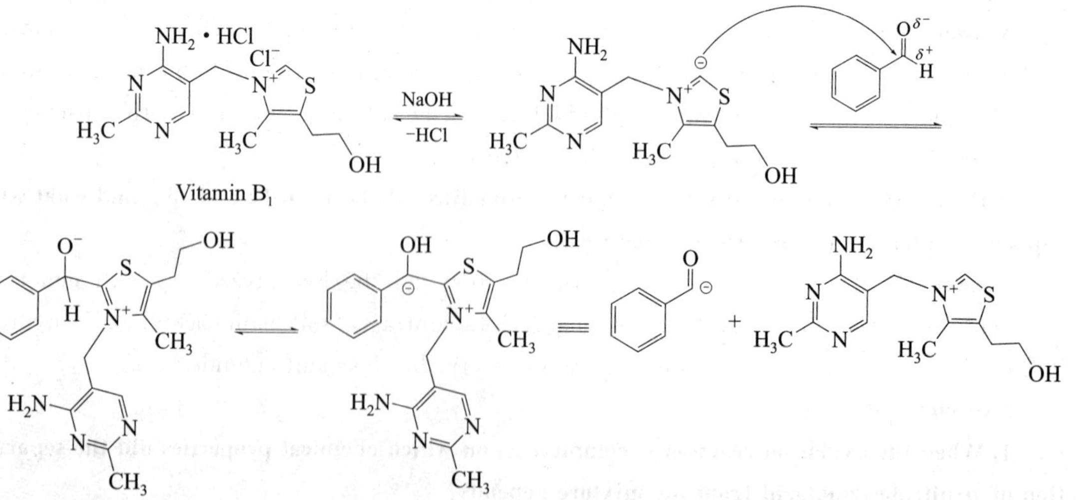

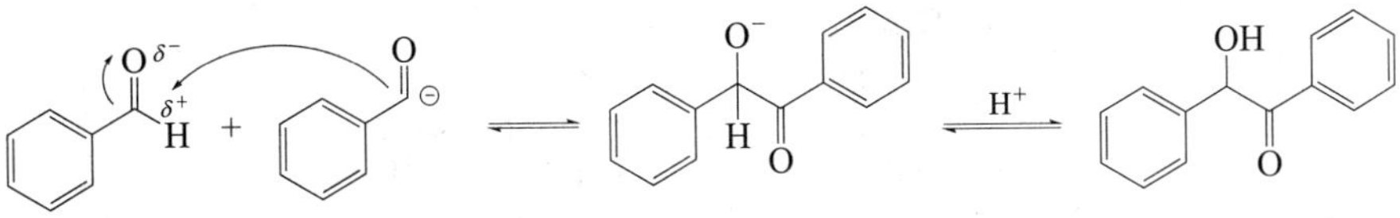

**2. Can benzoin be oxidized with concentrated nitric acid in the preparation of 1,2-diphenyl-ethylene ketone?**

**Answer:** No, strong oxidizers can destroy the chemical structure of benzoin and can not obtain the desired product.

**3. Structurally, explain the reaction mechanism for the formation of phenytoin.**

**Answer:**

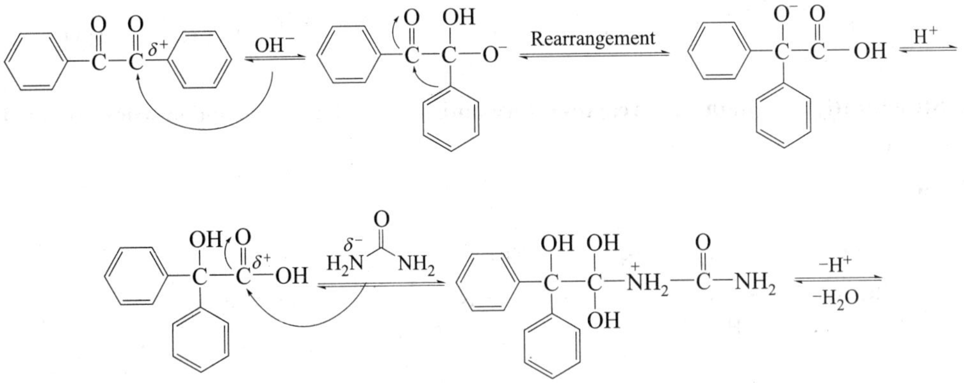

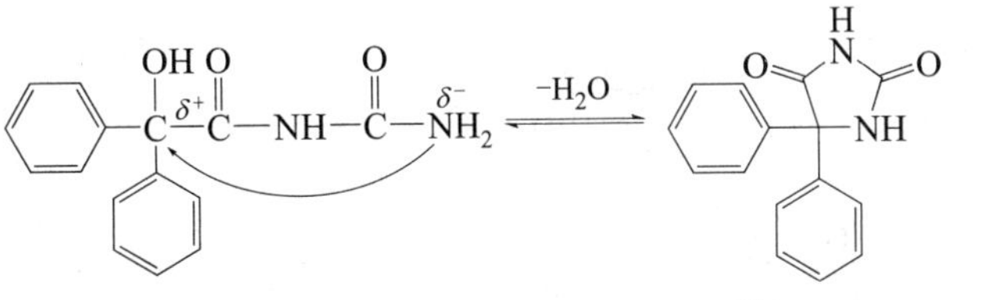

Phenytoin

**Experiment 9**

**1. Structurally, what substances can be used to replace triethylamine in the esterification reaction to produce neostigmine?**

**Answer:**

$$(CH_3CH_2CH_2)_2NH, \quad (CH_3CH_2CH_2)_3N,$$

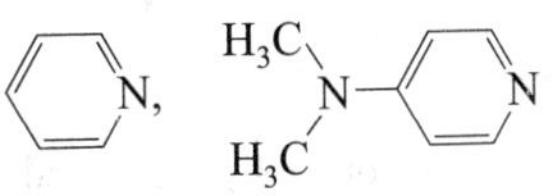

**2. Structurally, explain the reaction mechanism for the formation of neostigmine.**

**Answer:**

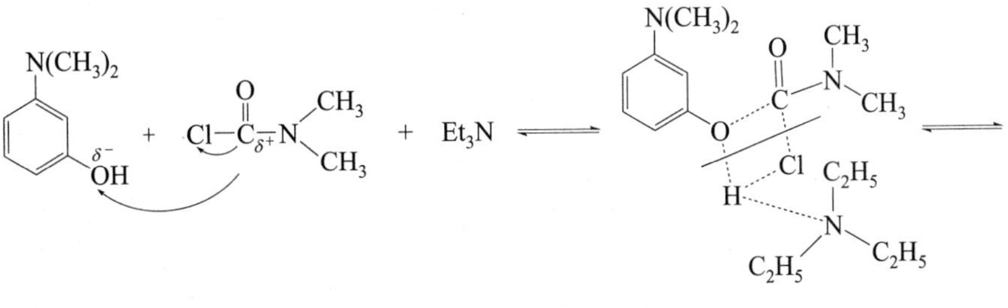

## Experiment 10

1. Structurally, why dose *p*-hydroxyacetophenone disssolve in potassium carbonate aqueous solution?

Answer:

$$HO-C_6H_4-COCH_3 + K_2CO_3 \longrightarrow {}^+K\text{-}O-C_6H_4-COCH_3 + CO_2\uparrow + H_2O$$

2. Structurally, explain the reaction mechanism of Mannich condensation to dyclonine hydrochlorid.

Answer:

Dyclonine hydrochlorid

# 附录二　思考题参考答案

**实验一**

1.作为脱色剂，活性炭为什么不能在沸腾时加入溶液中？

答：当溶液沸腾时，加入活性炭易引起暴沸，因此，加入活性炭时，需要将溶液稍微降温。

2.常用的重结晶溶剂有哪些？

答：水、氯仿、丙酮、乙酸乙酯、乙醇、甲醇，等。

**实验二**

1.用结构式表示，为什么在反应过程中室内会有醋酸的味道？

答：

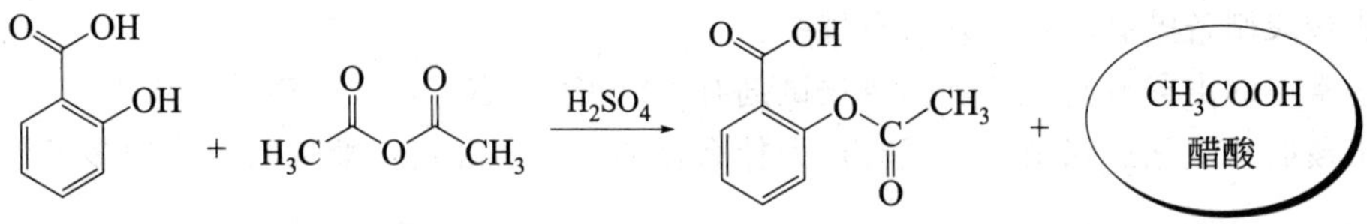

2.用结构式表示，为什么水杨酸和阿司匹林是酸性物质？

答：

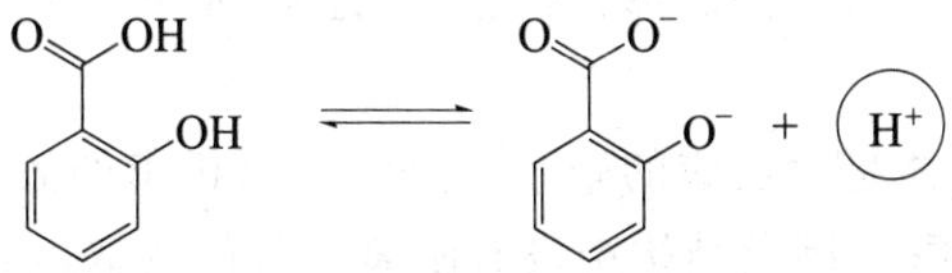

水杨酸

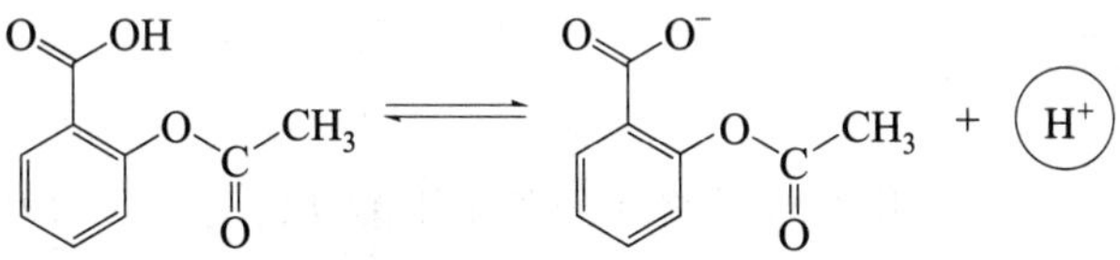

阿司匹林(2- 乙酰氧基苯甲酸)

**实验三**

1.本实验中乙酸可以作为乙酰化试剂来使用吗？

答：如果本实验用乙酸作用乙酰化试剂，反应时间将被延长，并且有很多副产物生成，产品纯度很差。

2.常见的乙酰化试剂有哪些？

答：常用的乙酰化试剂及它们的活性顺序如下：

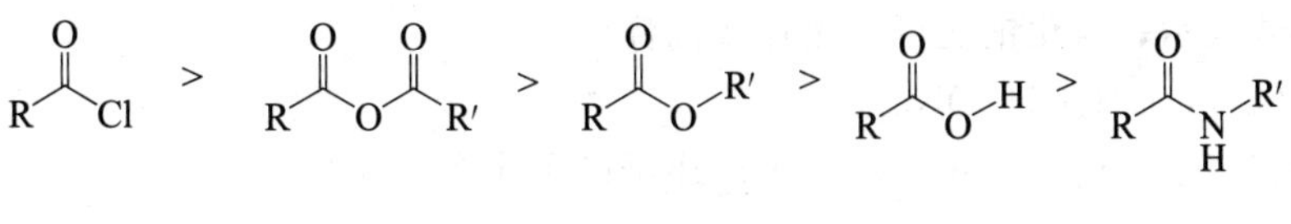

3. 合成扑热息痛时常见的杂质有哪些？

答：合成扑热息痛时常见的杂质有：

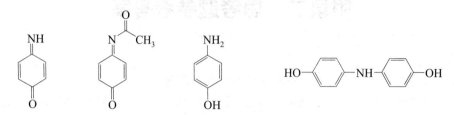

**实验四**

1. 为何不直接用阿司匹林和扑热息痛制备苯乐来？

答：阿司匹林是一种低活性的芳香酸，在吡啶的催化作用下和氯化亚砜反应可生成高活性的乙酰水杨酰氯。扑热息痛上酚羟基由于与苯环的共轭作用，其亲核性较弱，当变成钠盐后，其氧上的电子密度和亲核性都会增强，另外，碱化成盐后再与乙酰水杨酰氯反应可避免生成氯化氢。

2. 由羧酸制备酰氯的常用方法有哪些？

答：常用的由羧酸制备酰氯的氯化试剂有：$SOCl_2$，$(COCl)_2$，$PCl_3$，$PCl_5$。

3. 由羧酸和氯化亚砜制备酰氯时，为什么要加入少量吡啶？吡啶的量若加多了会发生什么后果？

答：吡啶可催化且加速反应的进行。吡啶过量时，会影响产品的质量和产量。

**实验五**

1. 反应过程中，pH＝7时析出的固体是什么？pH＝5时析出的固体是什么？在10％盐酸中的不溶物是什么？

答：pH＝7时析出的固体是为反应的磺胺；pH＝5时析出的固体是磺胺醋酰；在10％盐酸中的不溶物是磺胺双醋酰，因其结构中没有游离的芳伯胺基，故不能成盐析出。

2. 反应过程中，调节pH＝12～13是非常重要的，碱性过强或过弱会产生怎样的结果？

答：碱性过强，产物磺胺双醋酰、磺胺醋酰会水解，故磺胺较多；碱性过弱，磺胺双醋酰不易水解，磺胺较少。

**实验六**

1. 氧化反应完毕，依据哪些性质将对硝基苯甲酸从混合物中分离出来？

答：氧化反应以后，利用对硝基苯甲酸在酸性条件下不溶于水的特点，过滤保留固体除去水溶性杂质；碱性条件下，对硝基苯甲酸转化为对硝基苯基酸钠溶于水，过滤除去水不溶杂质；将滤液调酸以后，对硝基苯甲酸钠游离为对硝基苯甲酸后从水中析出，过滤要固体得到产品。

2. 酯化反应为什么需无水操作？

答：酯化反应是可逆反应，如果操作过程中有水，会导致原料不能反应完全，从而导致产率下降。

**实验七**

1. 用结构式表示，氢化钠还可以用什么代替？

答：$CH_3ONa$，$CH_3CH_2ONa$ 等。

2. 用结构式表示，所用 Lewis 酸 $ZnCl_2$ 还可以用什么代替？

答：$AlCl_3$，$BF_3 \cdot EtOEt$，$FeCl_3$，等。

3. 用结构式表示，所用异戊醇还可以用什么代替？

答：$CH_3CH_2CH_2CH_2CH_2OH$，$(CH_3)_3COH$，$CH_3CH_2CH_2CH_2OH$，等。

4. 哌嗪化反应时，6-氟发生哌嗪化的副产物的结构式是什么？

答：

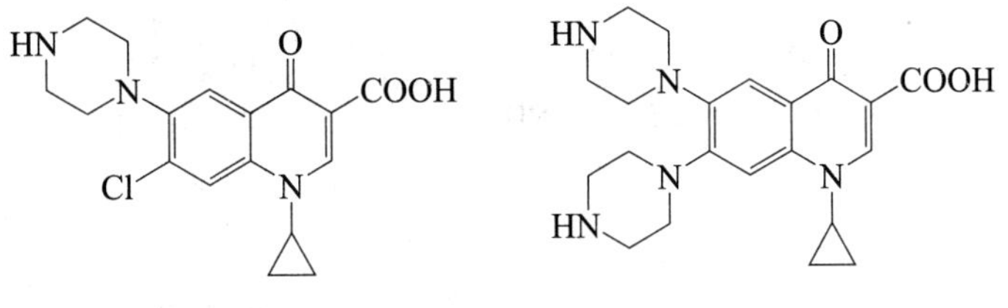

**实验八**

1. 用结构式表示维生素 $B_1$ 催化安息香缩合反应的机理。

答：

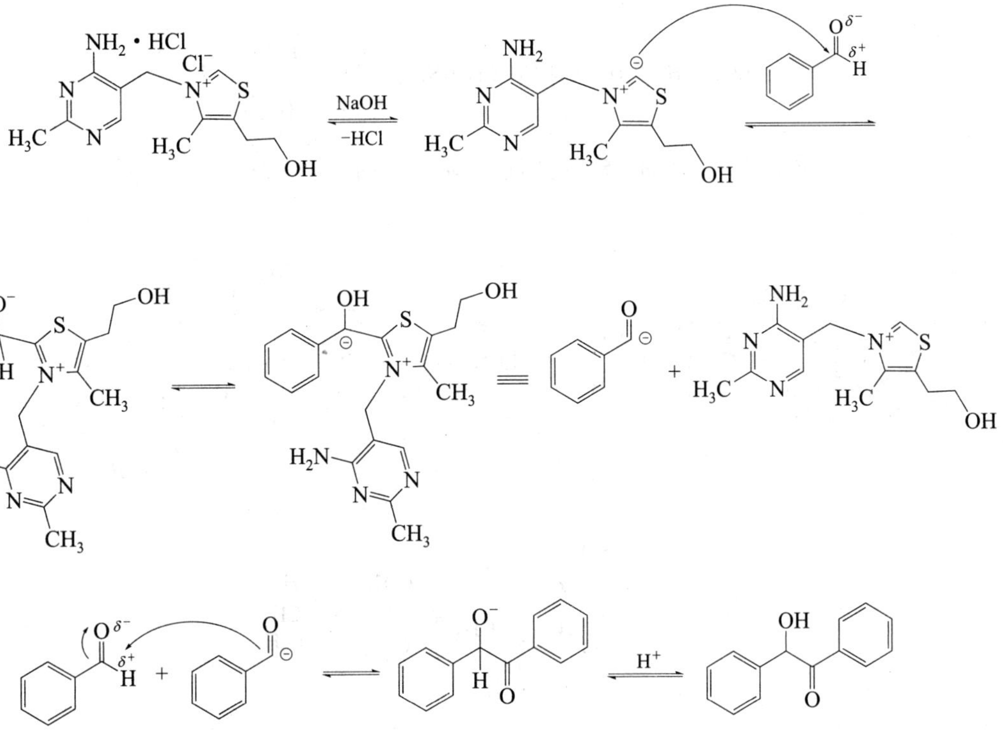

2. 在制备 1,2-二苯乙二酮时，能用浓硝酸氧化安息香吗？

答：不能，强氧化剂会破坏安息香化学结构，无法获得所需要产物。

3. 用结构式表示合成苯妥英这一步反应的反应机理？

答：

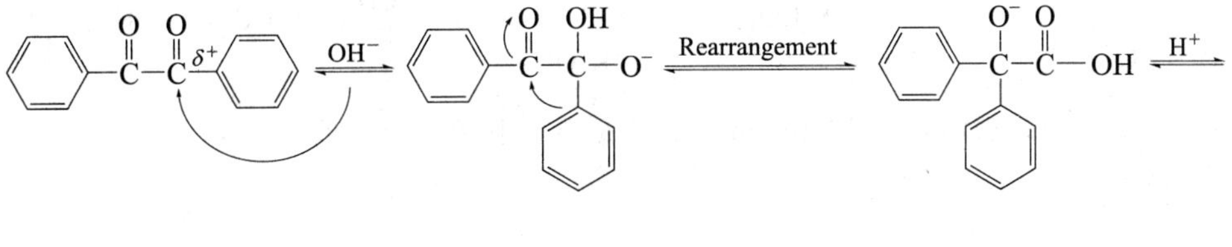

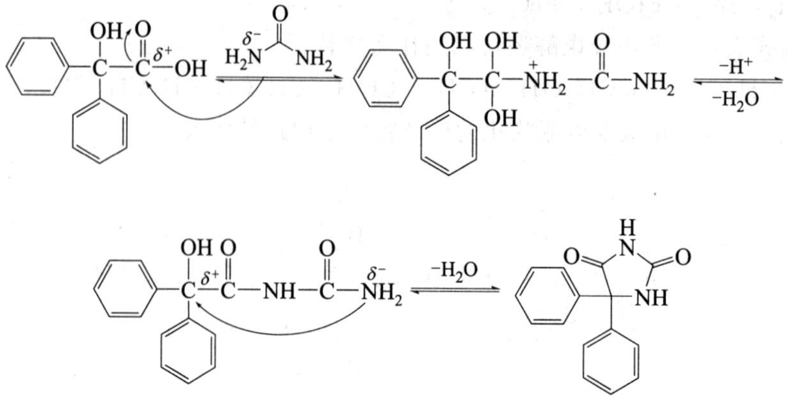

苯妥英

**实验九**

1.用结构式表示，酯化反应生成新斯的明时，可用什么物质取代三乙胺？

答：

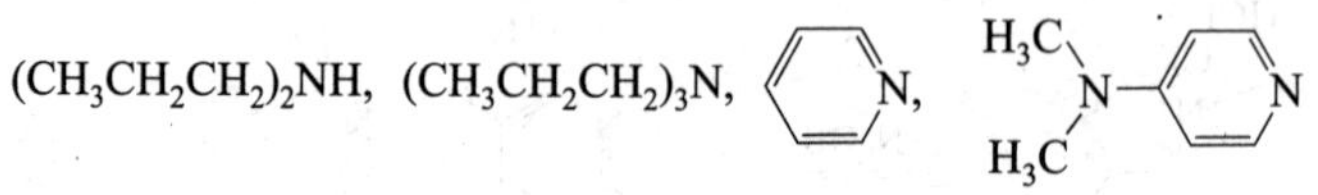

$(CH_3CH_2CH_2)_2NH$,  $(CH_3CH_2CH_2)_3N$,

2.用结构式表示，生成新斯的明这一步反应的反应机理。

答：

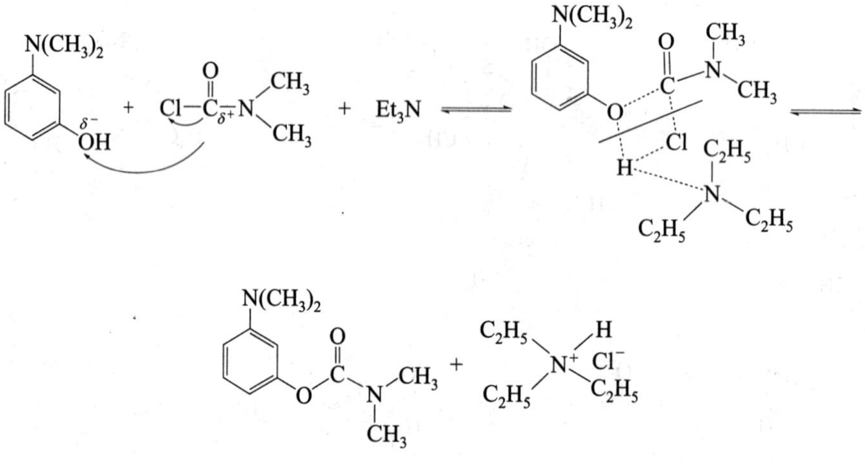

**实验十**

1.用结构式表示，为什么对羟基苯乙酮能溶于碳酸钾水溶液？

答：

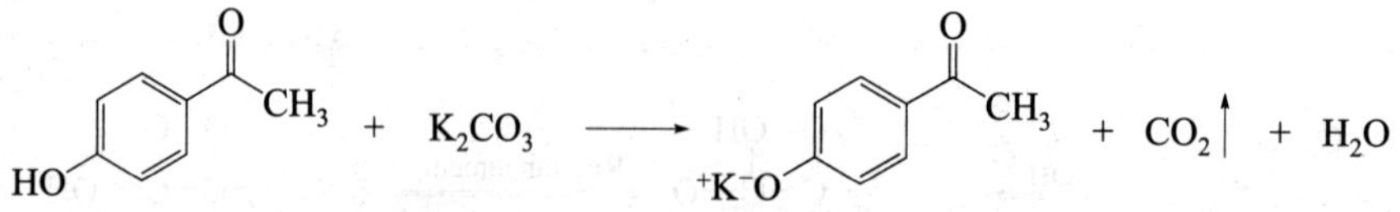

2.用结构式表示，经 Mannich 缩合生成盐酸达克罗宁的反应机理。

答：

盐酸达克罗宁

# Appendix 3　Common Instruments（常用仪器）

Beaker
烧杯

Round-bottom flask
圆底烧瓶

Three-necked round-bottom
三颈烧瓶

Erlenmeyer flask
锥形瓶

Filter flask
抽滤瓶

Buchner funnel
布氏漏斗

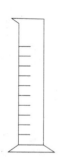

Graduated cylinder
量筒

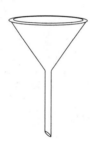

Glass funnel
玻璃漏斗

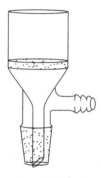

Glass filter funnel
玻璃砂芯漏斗

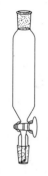

Dropping funnel
滴液漏斗

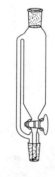

Constant pressure
dropping funnel
恒压滴液漏斗

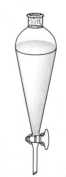

Separating funnel
分液漏斗

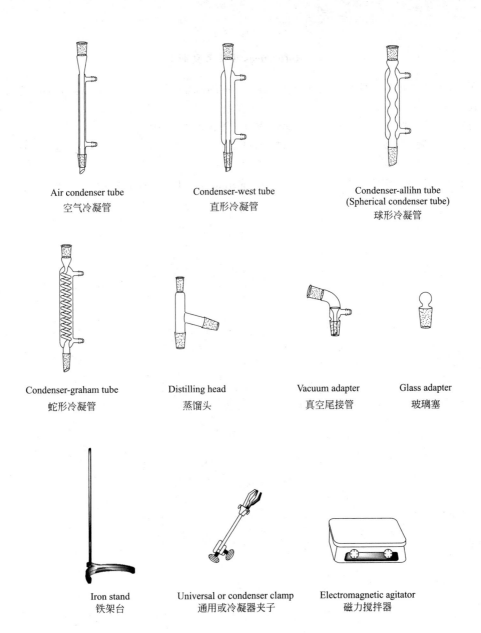

Air condenser tube
空气冷凝管

Condenser-west tube
直形冷凝管

Condenser-allihn tube
(Spherical condenser tube)
球形冷凝管

Condenser-graham tube
蛇形冷凝管

Distilling head
蒸馏头

Vacuum adapter
真空尾接管

Glass adapter
玻璃塞

Iron stand
铁架台

Universal or condenser clamp
通用或冷凝器夹子

Electromagnetic agitator
磁力搅拌器

# References（参考文献）

［1］ 尤启冬. 药物化学实验与指导（Experiment and medicinal chemistry）. 北京：中国医药科技出版社，2008.

［2］ 阿有梅，张红岭. 药物实验与指导，郑州：郑州大学出版社，2015.

［3］ 木合布力. 阿不力孜. 药物化学实验双语教程（Experiment of medicinal chemistry）. 北京：科学出版社，2016.

［4］ 马玉卓. 药物化学实验（Medicinal chemistry experiments）. 北京：科学出版社，2016.

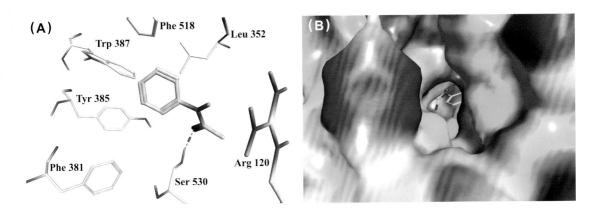

**Color Diagram 1** (A) The interaction model of acetanilide and COX-2 of cyclooxygenase (yellow represents acetanilide, white residue means cyclooxygenase COX-2); (B) Surface map of the binding site of acetanilide on COX-2 protein (hydrophobic interactions are shown in green, and acetanilide molecule and parts of the enzyme directly exposed to solvent are shown in yellow and red, respectively)

**彩插 1** （A）乙酰苯胺与环氧合酶COX-2的相互作用模式（黄色表示乙酰苯胺，白色残基表示环氧合酶COX-2）；（B）乙酰苯胺结合位点的表面图（绿色代表疏水性，红色代表蛋白直接暴露于溶剂）

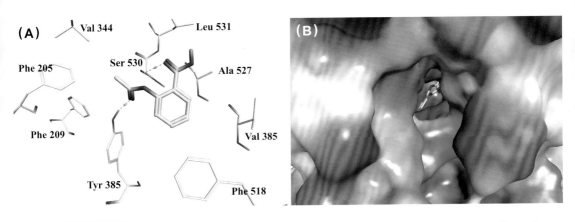

**Color Diagram 2** (A) Interaction patterns between aspirin and COX-2 (aspirin is shown in yellow whereas COX-2 amino acid residues are represented in white); (B) Surface map of the binding site of aspirin on COX-2 protein (hydrophobic interactions are shown in green, and aspirin molecule and parts of the enzyme directly exposed to solvent are shown in yellow and red, respectively)

**彩插 2** （A）阿司匹林与环氧合酶COX-2的相互作用模式（黄色表示阿司匹林，白色残基表示环氧合酶COX-2）；（B）阿司匹林结合位点的表面图（绿色代表疏水性，红色代表蛋白直接暴露于溶剂）

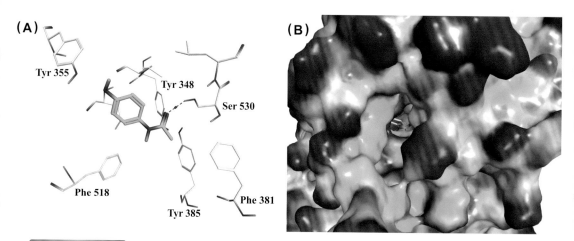

**Color Diagram 3** (A) Interaction of acetaminophen with COX-2 (green means acetaminophen, white means the residue of COX-2); (B) Surface map of acetaminophen binding sites on COX-2 protein (green represents hydrophobic, red represents the protein directly exposed to the solvent, yellow represents acetaminophen)

**彩插 3** （A）对乙酰氨基酚与COX-2的相互作用模式（绿色表示对乙酰氨基酚，白色残基为COX-2）；（B）对乙酰氨基酚结合位点的表面图（绿色代表疏水性，红色代表蛋白直接暴露于溶剂，黄色表示对乙酰氨基酚）

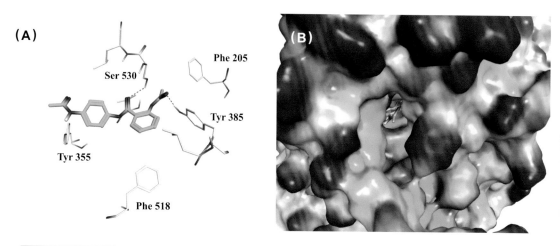

**Color Diagram 4** (A) Interaction patterns between benorilate and COX-2 (benorilate is shown in yellow whereas COX-2 amino acid residues are represented in white); (B) Surface map of the binding site of aspirin on COX-2 protein (hydrophobic interactions are shown in green, and benorilate molecule and parts of the enzyme directly exposed to solvent are shown in yellow and red, respectively)

**彩插 4** （A）苯乐来与COX-2的相互作用模式图（绿色表示苯乐来，白色残基为COX-2）；（B）苯乐来结合位点的表面图（绿色代表疏水性，红色代表蛋白直接暴露于溶剂，黄色代表苯乐来）

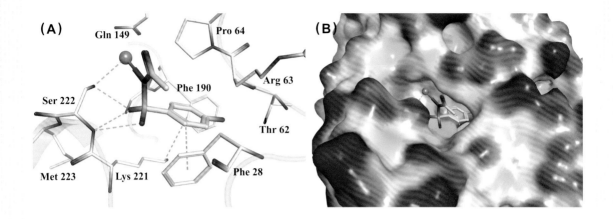

**Color Diagram 5** (A) Predicted binding mode of sulfacetamide sodium with dihydropteroate synthase (yellow for sulfacetamide sodium and white for important residues of dihydropteroate synthase); (B) The surface map of sulfacetamide sodium binding pocket of dihydropteroate synthase (green area represents hydrophobic regions and red area represents exposed region)

**彩插5** （A）磺胺醋酰钠与二氢叶酸合成酶的相互作用模式（黄色表示磺胺醋酰钠，白色残基表示二氢叶酸合成酶）；（B）磺胺醋酰钠结合位点的表面图（绿色代表疏水性，红色代表蛋白直接暴露于溶剂）

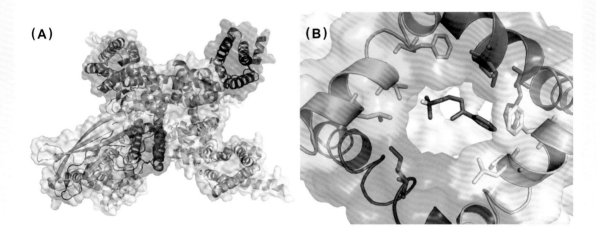

**Color Diagram 6** (A) Structure of the voltage-gated Na+ channel from electric eel; (B)Homology modeled structure of human voltage-gated Na+ channel in complex with benzocaine

**彩插6** （A）电鳗电压门控Na⁺通道的X衍射结构；（B）苯佐卡因与同源模建的人电压门控Na⁺通道的结合模式

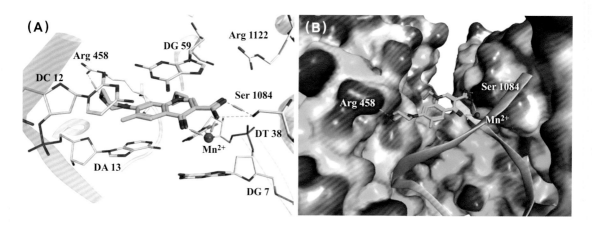

**Color Diagram 7** (A) The binding mode of ciprofloxacin with DNA gyrase (the residues of DNA gyrase and DNA bases are shown in white sticks and yellow sticks, respectively, hydrogen bonds are shown in green dash lines); (B) The protein surface of complex crystal structure of *Staphylococcus aureus* DNA gyrase with ciprofloxacin and DNA (hydrophobic region is green and solvent exposed region is red, DNA chains are yellow ribbons)

**彩插7** （A）环丙沙星与DNA回旋酶的结合模式图（与环丙沙星结合相关的DNA回旋酶残基和DNA碱基分别用白色和黄色棒状模型表示，氢键用绿色虚线表示）；（B）金黄色葡萄球菌DNA回旋酶、环丙沙星和DNA复合晶体蛋白表面图（疏水区域表示为绿色，溶剂暴露区域为红色，DNA链为黄色飘带）

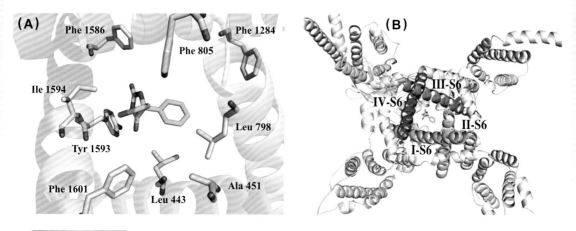

**Color Diagram 8** (A) The binding mode of phenytoin with VGSC (the key residues associated with phenytoin binding are shown in white sticks); (B) The protein surface of complex crystal structure of phenytoin with VGSC (VGSC is shown in cartoon ribbon, wherein the active site Ⅰ-S6 to Ⅳ-S6 segments are shown in green, yellow, orange, and magenta ribbons, respectively)

**彩插8** （A）苯妥英与VGSC结合模式图（与苯妥英结合相关的关键残基使用白色棒状模型表示）；（B）苯妥英与VGSC的结合模式表面图（VGSC以飘带表示，其中活性位点I-S6到Ⅳ-S6片段分别表示为绿色、黄色、橙色、洋红色飘带）

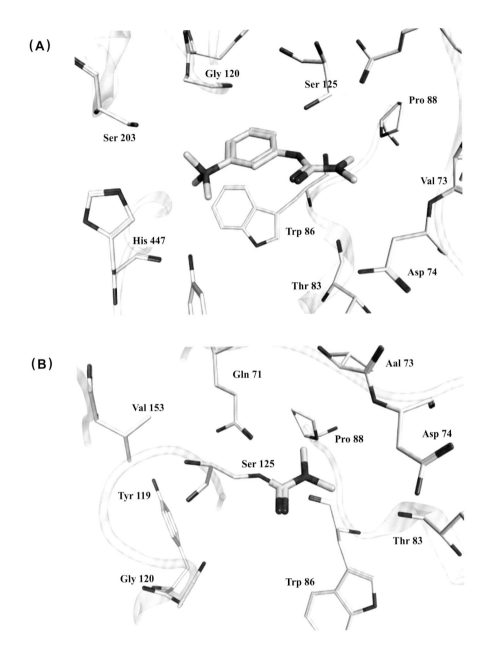

(A)

Gly 120

Ser 125

Pro 88

Ser 203

Val 73

His 447

Trp 86

Asp 74

Thr 83

(B)

Gln 71

Aal 73

Val 153

Pro 88

Asp 74

Ser 125

Tyr 119

Thr 83

Gly 120

Trp 86

**Color Diagram 9** The predicted binding model of neostigmine with AChE: (A) the complex of AChE with Neostigmine; (B)The predicted binding model of dimethylamino with AChE (the key residues associated with neostigmine binding are showed as white sticks)

**彩插9** 新斯的明在乙酰胆碱酯酶（PDB：6F25）中的预测结合模式（A）新斯的明-乙酰胆碱酯酶复合物；（B）二甲胺基甲酰化乙酰胆碱酯酶（与新斯的明结合的关键残基使用白色棒状模型表示）

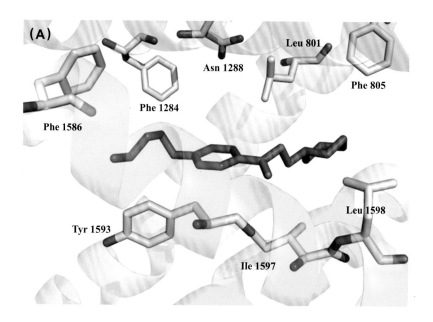

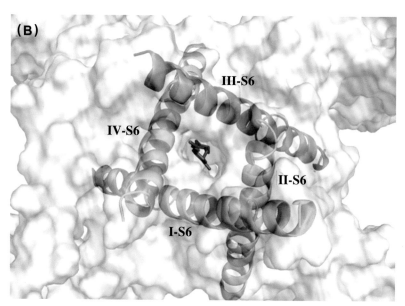

**Color Diagram 10** (A) The binding mode of dyclonine with VGSC (the key residues associated with dyclonine binding are shown in white sticks); (B)The protein surface of complex crystal structure of dyclonine with VGSC (VGSC is shown in cartoon ribbon, wherein the active site Ⅰ-S6 to Ⅳ-S6 segments are shown in green, yellow, orange, and cyan ribbons, respectively)

**彩插10** （A）达克罗宁在VGSC 活性位点的结合模式（VGSC 关键残基以白色棒状模型显示）；
（B）达克罗宁与VGSC的结合模式表面图（VGSC活性位点的I−S6到Ⅳ−S6片段分别用绿色、黄色、橙色、蓝绿色飘带表示）